D1388989

WS
804
CUR

Current Concepts in Neonatal Nutrition

Editors

BRENDA POINDEXTER
HEIDI KARPEN

CLINICS IN PERINATOLOGY

www.perinatology.theclinics.com

Consulting Editor
LUCKY JAIN

June 2014 • Volume 41 • Number 2

ELSEVIER

1600 John F. Kennedy Boulevard • Suite 1800 • Philadelphia, Pennsylvania, 19103-2899

http://www.theclinics.com

CLINICS IN PERINATOLOGY Volume 41, Number 2
June 2014 ISSN 0095-5108, ISBN-13: 978-0-323-29929-9

Editor: Kerry Holland
Developmental Editor: Casey Jackson

© **2014 Elsevier Inc. All rights reserved.**

This periodical and the individual contributions contained in it are protected under copyright by Elsevier, and the following terms and conditions apply to their use:

Photocopying

Single photocopies of single articles may be made for personal use as allowed by national copyright laws. Permission of the Publisher and payment of a fee is required for all other photocopying, including multiple or systematic copying, copying for advertising or promotional purposes, resale, and all forms of document delivery. Special rates are available for educational institutions that wish to make photocopies for non-profit educational classroom use. For information on how to seek permission visit www.elsevier.com/permissions or call: (+44) 1865 843830 (UK)/(+1) 215 239 3804 (USA).

Derivative Works

Subscribers may reproduce tables of contents or prepare lists of articles including abstracts for internal circulation within their institutions. Permission of the Publisher is required for resale or distribution outside the institution. Permission of the Publisher is required for all other derivative works, including compilations and translations (please consult www.elsevier.com/permissions).

Electronic Storage or Usage

Permission of the Publisher is required to store or use electronically any material contained in this periodical, including any article or part of an article (please consult www.elsevier.com/permissions). Except as outlined above, no part of this publication may be reproduced, stored in a retrieval system or transmitted in any form or by any means, electronic, mechanical, photocopying, recording or otherwise, without prior written permission of the Publisher.

Notice

No responsibility is assumed by the Publisher for any injury and/or damage to persons or property as a matter of products liability, negligence or otherwise, or from any use or operation of any methods, products, instructions or ideas contained in the material herein. Because of rapid advances in the medical sciences, in particular, independent verification of diagnoses and drug dosages should be made. Although all advertising material is expected to conform to ethical (medical) standards, inclusion in this publication does not constitute a guarantee or endorsement of the quality or value of such product or of the claims made of it by its manufacturer.

Clinics in Perinatology (ISSN 0095-5108) is published quarterly by Elsevier Inc., 360 Park Avenue South, New York, NY 10010-1710. Months of issue are March, June, September, and December. Business and Editorial Offices: 1600 John F. Kennedy Blvd., Ste. 1800, Philadelphia, PA 19103-2899. Customer Service Office: 3251 Riverport Lane, Maryland Heights, MO 63043. Periodicals postage paid at New York, NY and additional mailing offices. Subscription prices are $285.00 per year (US individuals), $445.00 per year (US institutions), $340.00 per year (Canadian individuals), $545.00 per year (Canadian institutions), $420.00 per year (foreign individuals), $545.00 per year (foreign institutions), $135.00 per year (US students), and $195.00 per year (Canadian and foreign students). Foreign air speed delivery is included in all Clinics subscription prices. All prices are subject to change without notice. **POSTMASTER:** Send address changes to *Clinics in Perinatology*, Elsevier Health Sciences Division, Subscription Customer Service, 3251 Riverport Lane, Maryland Heights, MO 63043. **Customer Service: Telephone: 1-800-654-2452** (U.S. and Canada); **1-314-447-8871** (outside U.S. and Canada). **Fax: 1-314-447-8029. E-mail: journalscustomerservice-usa@elsevier.com** (for print support); **journalsonlinesupport-usa@elsevier.com** (for online support).

Reprints. For copies of 100 or more, of articles in this publication, please contact the Commercial Reprints Department, Elsevier Inc., 360 Park Avenue South, New York, NY 10010-1710. Tel. 212-633-3874; Fax: 212-633-3820; E-mail: reprints@elsevier.com.

Clinics in Perinatology is also pubilshed in Spanish by McGraw-Hill Interamericana Editores S.A., P.O. Box 5-237, 06500 Mexico D.F., Mexico.

Clinics in Perinatology is covered in *MEDLINE/PubMed (Index Medicus) Current Contents, Excepta Medica, BIOSIS and ISI/BIOMED.*

Printed in the United States of America.

Contributors

CONSULTING EDITOR

LUCKY JAIN, MD, MBA
Richard W. Blumberg Professor and Executive Vice Chairman, Department of Pediatrics, Emory University School of Medicine; Executive Medical Director, Children's Physician Group, Emory Children's Center, Children's Healthcare of Atlanta, Atlanta, Georgia

EDITORS

BRENDA POINDEXTER, MD
Associate Professor of Clinical Pediatrics, Department of Pediatrics, Riley Hospital for Children at Indiana University Health, Indianapolis, Indiana

HEIDI KARPEN, MD
Assistant Professor, Department of Pediatrics, Emory University School of Medicine, Children's Healthcare of Atlanta, Atlanta, Georgia

AUTHORS

STEVEN A. ABRAMS, MD
US Department of Agriculture/Agriculture Research Service, Department of Pediatrics, Children's Nutrition Research Center, Texas Children's Hospital, Baylor College of Medicine, Houston, Texas

DAVID H. ADAMKIN, MD
Director, Division of Neonatal Medicine; Professor of Pediatrics; University of Louisville School of Medicine, Louisville, Kentucky

LAURA D. BROWN, MD
Section of Neonatology, Department of Pediatrics, Anschutz Medical Campus, University of Colorado School of Medicine, Aurora, Colorado

KARA L. CALKINS, MD
Division of Neonatology and Developmental Biology, Department of Pediatrics, Mattel Children's Hospital, Assistant Clinical Professor, University of California, Los Angeles, Los Angeles, California

REESE H. CLARK, MD
The Center for Research, Education, and Quality, MEDNAX Services/Pediatrix Medical Group/American Anesthesiology, Sunrise, Florida

TARAH T. COLAIZY, MD, MPH
Associate Professor of Pediatrics; Carver College of Medicine, University of Iowa, Iowa City, Iowa

PATRICIA W. DENNING, MD
Associate Professor, Division of Neonatology, Department of Pediatrics, Emory University School of Medicine, Atlanta, Georgia

SHERIN U. DEVASKAR, MD
Division of Neonatology and Developmental Biology, Department of Pediatrics, Mattel Children's Hospital, Distinguished Professor, University of California, Los Angeles, Los Angeles, California

KIMBERLY L. DINH, PharmD
Clinical Pharmacy Specialist, Neonatal Intensive Care, Texas Children's Hospital, Houston, Texas

RICHARD A. EHRENKRANZ, MD
Professor of Pediatrics & Interim Chief; Section of Neonatal-Perinatal Medicine, Department of Neonatal-Perinatal Medicine, Yale University School of Medicine, New Haven, Connecticut

KELI M. HAWTHORNE, MS, RD
Senior Registered Dietitian, US Department of Agriculture/Agriculture Research Service, Department of Pediatrics, Children's Nutrition Research Center, Texas Children's Hospital, Baylor College of Medicine, Houston, Texas

WILLIAM W. HAY Jr, MD
Section of Neonatology, Department of Pediatrics, Anschutz Medical Campus, University of Colorado School of Medicine, Aurora, Colorado

KENDRA HENDRICKSON, MS, RD, CNSC, CSP
Department of Food & Nutrition, Anschutz Medical Campus, University of Colorado Hospital, Aurora, Colorado

BRETT M. JAKAITIS, MD
Fellow, Division of Neonatology, Department of Pediatrics, Emory University School of Medicine, Atlanta, Georgia

MARIA MAKRIDES, RD, PhD
Healthy Mothers, Babies and Children, South Australian Health and Medical Research Institute, Adelaide; Women's and Children's Health Research Institute, University of Adelaide, North Adelaide, South Australia, Australia

CAMILIA R. MARTIN, MD, MS
Associate Director, NICU, Department of Neonatology; Director for Cross-Disciplinary Research Partnerships; Assistant Professor of Pediatrics; Division of Translational Research, Beth Israel Deaconess Medical Center, Harvard Medical School, Boston, Massachusetts

MARC L. MASOR, PhD
Science Educator; Former Director, Clinical Nutrition Research, Abbott Nutrition, Durango, Colorado

NNEKA I. NZEGWU, DO
Fellow, Neonatal-Perinatal Medicine, Department of Pediatrics, Section of Neonatal-Perinatal Medicine, Yale University School of Medicine, New Haven, Connecticut

IRENE E. OLSEN, PhD, RD, LDN
School of Nursing, University of Pennsylvania, Philadelphia, Pennsylvania

KATIE M. PFISTER, MD
Division of Neonatology, Department of Pediatrics, University of Minnesota, Minneapolis, Minnesota

JENNIFER L. PLACENCIA, PharmD
Clinical Pharmacy Specialist, Neonatal Intensive Care, Texas Children's Hospital, Houston, Texas

PAULA G. RADMACHER, MSPH, PhD
Research Manager; Assistant Professor, Neonatal Nutrition Research Laboratory, University of Louisville School of Medicine, Louisville, Kentucky

SARA E. RAMEL, MD
Division of Neonatology, Department of Pediatrics, University of Minnesota, Minneapolis, Minnesota

ALAN R. SPITZER, MD
Senior Vice President for Research, Education, and Quality; MEDNAX Services/Pediatrix Medical Group/American Anesthesiology, Sunrise, Florida

BONNIE E. STEPHENS, MD
Adjunct Assistant Professor of Pediatrics; Warren Alpert Medical School, Brown University, Providence, Rhode Island; Medical Director, NICU, Community Medical Center, Missoula, Montana

RICARDO UAUY, MD, PhD
Division of Neonatology, Department of Pediatrics, Catholic University Medical School and Institute of Nutrition, INTA University of Chile, Santiago, Chile

ROBERT S. VENICK, MD
Division of Gastroenterology, Department of Pediatrics, Mattel Children's Hospital, Associate Clinical Professor, University of California, Los Angeles, Los Angeles, California

BETTY R. VOHR, MD
Director, Neonatal Follow-up Program, Women and Infants Hospital; Professor of Pediatrics, Warren Alpert Medical School, Brown University, Providence, Rhode Island

Contents

> The concept that adequate nutritional status and normal growth are important is well-accepted. How to assess the adequacy of nutrition and how to define appropriate growth remains an area of active debate. Our goal is to review how growth is assessed at birth and during the hospital stay of prematurely born infants, and to offer a standardized approach.

> Despite advances in care, preterm infants exhibit disproportionate growth and neurodevelopmental delay attributable to both nutritional and nonnutritional factors. These infants have prolonged linear stunting and decreased fat-free mass compared with their term counterparts. These 2 metrics index organ growth and development (including the brain) and protein accretion. Protein, along with carbohydrates, fats, and zinc, plays key roles in brain development, and deficiencies can lead to linear growth failure, abnormalities in the growth hormone axis, and developmental delay. Optimization of nutrition, including protein intake, decreasing inflammatory episodes, and enhancing the growth hormone axis will likely improve long-term outcomes.

> There is a compelling body of literature that suggests that the provision of an inadequate amount of protein to preterm infants in the neonatal period has detrimental effects on the developing brain with the potential to result in long-term, neurodevelopmental sequelae. Although a great deal of indirect evidence implies that the provision of adequate amounts of protein may be associated with better neurodevelopmental outcomes, there remains a paucity of direct evidence that would allow us to draw any final conclusions.

> Although parenteral nutrition (PN) is life-sustaining, it is associated with many complications including parenteral nutrition–associated liver disease (PNALD) and central line–associated bloodstream infections (CLABSIs), which carry a high morbidity and mortality and impose a burden on the health care system. Evidence has emerged that the dose and composition

of intravenous lipid products may alter the incidence of PNALD. However, other patient and PN-related factors, such as prematurity, birth weight, and gastrointestinal anatomy and function, are important. To improve neonatal care, future research on optimizing the content of PN and decreasing the incidence IFALD and CLABSIs is required.

Micronutrient requirements are well-established for healthy full-term infants. However, few such recommendations exist for high-risk infants, including full-term infants with a variety of medical disorders or very preterm infants. Key micronutrients considered in this review are calcium, phosphorus, magnesium, iron, and zinc. The ongoing unresolved shortages, especially of intravenous forms of these minerals, remain a major problem. Considered are some aspects of how the nutrient shortages may be managed, recognizing the complexity and changing nature of the supply.

Challenges remain in optimizing the delivery of fatty acids to attain their nutritional and therapeutic benefits in neonatal health. In this review, knowledge about placental transfer of fatty acids to the developing fetus is summarized, the potential role and mechanisms of fatty acids in enhancing neonatal health and minimizing morbidities is outlined, the unique considerations for fatty acid delivery in the preterm population are defined, and the research questions are proposed that need to be addressed before new standards of care are adopted at the bedside for the provision of critical fatty acids to preterm infants.

Relatively high amounts of protein are required to achieve normal fractional protein synthetic rates during the late second through early third trimester of fetal growth. Once preterm infants achieve higher protein intakes for sustained periods, growth begins to approximate that of the normally growing fetus and long-term neurodevelopmental outcomes are improved. Preterm formulas have been developed that are enriched in protein. This review discusses several factors when using standard preterm formulas and high-protein preterm formulas in the neonatal intensive care unit, with an emphasis on quantity and quality of enteral protein delivery and risks to insufficient and/or excess protein administration.

The American Academy of Pediatrics supports the feeding of human milk for all infants. Very-low-birth-weight and extremely low-birth-weight infants especially can benefit from the immune and neurodevelopmental effects of human milk. However, human milk alone is nutritionally inadequate for the rapid growth of the very-low-birth-weight infant during a critical window for brain development and requires fortification to meet current recommendations. There are a variety of products, devices, and strategies that can be used to fine tune nutritional support of these very vulnerable infants.

goal of nutrition in these preterm infants is to match the intrauterine growth curves of the normally growing fetus. Despite this recommendation from the American Academy of Pediatrics Committee on Nutrition, neonatologists struggle daily to meet this goal, and as a result, postnatal growth failure and restriction are common. This article reviews post-discharge nutrition in the VLBW population, examining different types of post-discharge nutrition, current evidence, and future and remaining questions. In addition, recommendations are provided for post-discharge nutrition in this population.

PROGRAM OBJECTIVE

The goal of *Clinics in Perinatology* is to keep practicing perinatologists, neonatologists, obstetricians, practicing physicians and residents up to date with current clinical practice in perinatology by providing timely articles reviewing the state of the art in patient care.

TARGET AUDIENCE

Perinatologists, neonatologists, obstetricians, practicing physicians, residents and healthcare professionals who provide patient care utilizing findings from *Clinics in Perinatology*.

LEARNING OBJECTIVES

Upon completion of this activity, participants will be able to:
1. Discuss the use of donor human milk and the use of high protein formulas in preterm infants.
2. Recognize the nutritional needs of low birth weight and very low birth weight infants.
3. Review the fatty acid requirements in preterm infant health and disease.

ACCREDITATION

The Elsevier Office of Continuing Medical Education (EOCME) is accredited by the Accreditation Council for Continuing Medical Education (ACCME) to provide continuing medical education for physicians.

The EOCME designates this enduring material for a maximum of 15 *AMA PRA Category 1 Credit*(s)™. Physicians should claim only the credit commensurate with the extent of their participation in the activity.

All other health care professionals requesting continuing education credit for this enduring material will be issued a certificate of participation.

DISCLOSURE OF CONFLICTS OF INTEREST

The EOCME assesses conflict of interest with its instructors, faculty, planners, and other individuals who are in a position to control the content of CME activities. All relevant conflicts of interest that are identified are thoroughly vetted by EOCME for fair balance, scientific objectivity, and patient care recommendations. EOCME is committed to providing its learners with CME activities that promote improvements or quality in healthcare and not a specific proprietary business or a commercial interest.

The planning committee, staff, authors and editors listed below have identified no financial relationships or relationships to products or devices they or their spouse/life partner have with commercial interest related to the content of this CME activity:

Steven A. Abrams, MD; David H. Adamkin, MD; Laura D. Brown, MD; Kara Lynne Calkins, MD; Reese H. Clark, MD; Tarah T. Colaizy, MD, MPH; Patricia Denning, MD; Sherin U. Devaskar, MD; Kimberly L. Dinh, PharmD; Richard A. Ehrenkranz, MD; Keli M. Hawthorne, MS, RD; William W. Hay. Jr, MD; Kendra Hendrickson, MS, RD, CNSC, CSP; Kerry Holland; Brynne Hunter; Brett M. Jakaitis, MD; Heidi Karpen, MD; Marc L. Masor, PhD; Jill McNair; Palani Murugesan; Nneka I. Nzegwu, DO; Irene E. Olsen, PhD, RD, LDN; Lindsay Parnell; Katie M. Pfister, MD; Jennifer L. Placencia, PharmD; Brenda B. Poindexter, MD; Paula G. Radmacher, MSPH, PhD; Sara E. Ramel, MD; Bonnie E. Stephens, MD; Robert S. Venick, MD; Betty R. Vohr, MD.

The planning committee, staff, authors and editors listed below have identified financial relationships or relationships to products or devices they or their spouse/life partner have with commercial interest related to the content of this CME activity:

Maria Makrides, RD, PhD; is a consultant/advisor for Nestle Health Science Scientific Advisory Board, Fonterra Cooperative Group Scientific Advisory Board and Nutricia Scientific Advisory Board; has research grants from National Health and Medical Research Council and Mead Johnson & Company, LLC. Camilia R. Martin, MD, MS; is a consultant/advisor for Mead Johnson & Company, LLC, Nestle Health Science and Alcresta; has research grants from Abbott Laboratories Nutritionals and Alcresta.
Alan R. Spitzer, MD; has stock ownership and employment affiliation with Mednax; has royalties/patents with Elsevier.
Ricardo Uauy, MD, PhD; has research grants from Fondecyt Chile, National Institutes of Health, World Cancer Research Fund International and Wellcome Trust UK.

UNAPPROVED/OFF-LABEL USE DISCLOSURE

The EOCME requires CME faculty to disclose to the participants:
1. When products or procedures being discussed are off-label, unlabelled, experimental, and/or investigational (not US Food and Drug Administration (FDA) approved); and

2. Any limitations on the information presented, such as data that are preliminary or that represent ongoing research, interim analyses, and/or unsupported opinions. Faculty may discuss information about pharmaceutical agents that is outside of FDA-approved labelling. This information is intended solely for CME and is not intended to promote off-label use of these medications. If you have any questions, contact the medical affairs department of the manufacturer for the most recent prescribing information.

TO ENROLL
To enroll in the *Clinics in Perinatology* Continuing Medical Education program, call customer service at 1-800-654-2452 or sign up online at http://www.theclinics.com/home/cme. The CME program is available to subscribers for an additional annual fee of $235 USD.

METHOD OF PARTICIPATION
In order to claim credit, participants must complete the following:
1. Complete enrolment as indicated above.
2. Read the activity.
3. Complete the CME Test and Evaluation. Participants must achieve a score of 70% on the test. All CME Tests and Evaluations must be completed online.

CME INQUIRIES/SPECIAL NEEDS
For all CME inquiries or special needs, please contact elsevierCME@elsevier.com.

CLINICS IN PERINATOLOGY

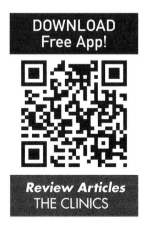

DOWNLOAD
Free App!

Review Articles
THE CLINICS

NOW AVAILABLE FOR YOUR iPhone and iPad

Foreword

Our Babies Are What We Feed Them

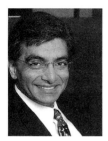

Lucky Jain, MD, MBA
Consulting Editor

"*Tell me what you eat and I will tell you what you are*," so wrote Anthelme Brillat-Savarin nearly 300 years ago.[1] This age-old saying can be extrapolated to our NICUs to mean, "*Tell me how you feed your babies and I will tell you how well you care for them*." Indeed, generations can be impacted by small changes in feeding practices early in life. *If we are what we eat, then our babies are what we feed them!*

Managing nutritional needs of sick neonates has never been easy. When choices lie between optimizing heart and lung function of a sick neonate versus advancing nutrition, nutrition often takes the back seat. The result is a nutritional deficit that accrues in the first weeks of life and is often hard to overcome in subsequent weeks (**Fig. 1**). The goal for nutrition of the preterm infant should be to get to the same growth rate a normal fetus would have achieved at the same gestational age in utero. Mother's milk would be optimal but is often not available. Poor gut motility, reflux, and inadequate digestive function further complicate the picture. The cause of postnatal growth restriction in preterm infants is arguably multifactorial, but it has been estimated that about 50% of the variance can be attributed to inadequate nutrition.[2] There is also a delicate balance between optimizing caloric intake and running the risk of complications such as fluid overload, liver damage, and necrotizing enterocolitis (NEC). The result: an unacceptable level of variability in practices and outcomes when it comes to growth and nutrition.

Yet there are solutions.[3] Breast milk has been shown to have innumerable benefits but is still grossly underutilized. It is not always clear why that is the case; socioeconomic status and lack of maternal commitment have often been blamed but many inner-city NICUs claim near universal breast-feeding rates. Numerous studies have shown that breast milk is better tolerated and reduces the risk of NEC. There are also immunologic benefits that translate to lower risk of infections and immune disorders later on in life.

Then there is the issue of early and aggressive versus delayed and slow feeding advances. Evidence shows that early initiation and targeted rapid advances result in

Clin Perinatol 41 (2014) xv–xvii
http://dx.doi.org/10.1016/j.clp.2014.04.001
0095-5108/14/$ – see front matter © 2014 Elsevier Inc. All rights reserved.

perinatology.theclinics.com

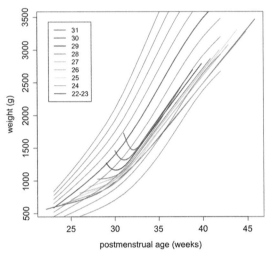

Fig. 1. Mean growth curves of weight by postmenstrual age and week of gestation, superimposed on the British 1990 birth weight reference. (*Adapted from* Cole TJ, Statnikov Y, Santhakumaran S, et al. Birth weight and longitudinal growth in infants born below 32 weeks' gestation: a UK population study. Arch Dis Child Fetal Neonatal Ed 2014;99:F38; with permission.)

better feeding tolerance and enhanced growth[4]; yet, few neonatologists take advantage of the fact that the fetus actively swallows amniotic fluid in large quantities throughout gestation and is, as such, adept at enteral feeds. Lack of early enteral feeds has its consequences with total parenteral nutrition–induced complications and slower acceptance of feeds later on. Introducing progressive enteral feeds before 4 days after birth in very low-birth-weight infants and advancing the rate of feed volumes at more than 24 mL/kg/d do not increase the risk of NEC.[5]

There are clearly many more issues that could benefit from open discussion and consensus-driven practices, particularly where evidence-based guidance is lacking. As Drs Poindexter and Karpen point out in their preface, this is an exciting time in neonatal nutrition with a "shift in focus from just survival and growth to optimizing the effect of each micro/macronutrient on long-term development and disease prevention."

I am delighted that Drs Poindexter and Karpen have put together a comprehensive review of advances in neonatal nutrition in this edition of the *Clinics in Perinatology*. In addition to the authors, I would like to thank Kerry Holland and her team at Elsevier for their support of this important topic. As Adelle Davis[2] pointed out in a *Time* article several years ago, the consequences of our feeding choices are stark: "*every day you do one of two things: build health or produce disease.*" Nowhere is this statement truer than in our NICUs.

Lucky Jain, MD, MBA
Emory University School of Medicine
Children's Healthcare of Atlanta
2015 Uppergate Drive
Atlanta, GA 30322, USA

E-mail address:
ljain@emory.edu

REFERENCES

1. Swanson PD. We are what we eat. Gastronomica J Crit Food Stud 2012. April 13, Web Exclusives.
2. Corpeleijin WE, Kouwenhoven SM, van Goudoever JB. Optimal growth of preterm infants. World Rev Nutr Diet 2013;106:149–55.
3. Hay WW. Strategies for feeding the preterm infant. Neonatology 2008;94:245–54.
4. Morgan J, Young L, McGuire W. Slow advancement of enteral feed volumes to prevent necrotizing enterocolitis in very low birth weight infants. Cochrane Database Syst Rev 2013;(3):CD001241.
5. The SIFT Investigators Group. Early enteral feeding strategies for very preterm infants: current evidence from Cochrane reviews. Arch Dis Child Fetal Neonatal Ed 2013;98:F470–2.

Preface

Neonatal Nutrition

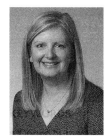 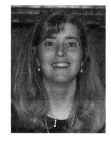

Brenda Poindexter, MD   Heidi Karpen, MD
Editors

Over the past several decades, advances in neonatal nutrition have focused on the provision of early parenteral nutrition and the development of formulas and supplements that most closely approximate maternal breast milk. The overall outcomes for infants, including premature infants, have greatly benefited from these advances, but there are still many nutritional unknowns that impact the lives of neonates. This is an exciting time in neonatal nutrition as the focus has shifted from survival and growth, which are still important goals, to effects of each micro/macronutrient on development, prevention of disease states such as ROP, the effects of neonatal nutrition on future health as an adult, and opportunities to improve long-term neurodevelopmental outcomes by optimal early nutrition.

This issue focuses on aspects of enteral and parenteral nutrition that are at the forefront of neonatal care: assessing growth, parenteral nutrition components (including alternate lipid formulations), optimal storage and use of human milk (including donor milk), post-discharge nutrition, and the effects of various micro/macronutrients on long-term developmental outcomes. It is anticipated that the study and implementation of many of these novel concepts into the care of neonates, many of whom are severely premature, will be of value to practitioners, researchers, and, most of all, our patients.

Brenda Poindexter, MD
Riley Hospital for Children
at Indiana University Health
Department of Pediatrics
Indiana University School of Medicine
699 Riley Hospital Drive RR208
Room 5900
Indianapolis, IN 46202, USA

E-mail address:
bpoindex@iu.edu (B. Poindexter)

Heidi Karpen, MD
Emory University School of Medicine
Children's Healthcare of Atlanta
Department of Pediatrics
2105 Uppergate Drive NE, Room 324
Atlanta, GA 30033, USA

E-mail address:
hkarpen@emory.edu (H. Karpen)

Clin Perinatol 41 (2014) xix
http://dx.doi.org/10.1016/j.clp.2014.03.001
0095-5108/14/$ – see front matter © 2014 Published by Elsevier Inc.

perinatology.theclinics.com

Assessment of Neonatal Growth in Prematurely Born Infants

Reese H. Clark, MD[a,*], Irene E. Olsen, PhD, RD, LDN[b],
Alan R. Spitzer, MD[a]

KEYWORDS

- Growth assessment • Neonatal growth • Premature infants • Body proportionality
- Growth curves • Small for gestational age • Growth status

KEY POINTS

- Growth assessment should start at birth and continue on weekly intervals at a minimum thereafter; birth and weekly assessments should include weight, length, and head circumference.
- Assigning an infant a set of percentiles for weight, length, and head circumference at birth provides an estimate of morbidity risk and target goals for growth.
- Where an infant's growth measurements plot on growth charts and the assignment of specific growth measurement percentiles differs between each set of charts. Assessment of change in size over time, however, is comparable between growth charts.
- Monitoring growth on growth curves allows for intervention when it decreases from birth percentiles; in this setting, precise percentile measurements are less important than the pattern of growth over time.
- Because body composition is not routinely measured in the neonatal intensive care unit, a proxy, such as body mass index, may be a useful clinical tool for preterm infants.

INTRODUCTION

The assessment and surveillance of growth in infants and children is recognized as an important part of health assessment.[1,2] Many disturbances in health and nutrition, independent of their etiology, alter growth. The goals of monitoring growth are to improve nutritional status, reduce the risk of inadequate nutritional intake, educate caregivers, and produce early detection and evaluation of conditions manifested by growth disorders. Understanding inadequate growth and excess growth are both important. The focus of this review, therefore, is the examination and evaluation of optimal growth in prematurely born infants.

[a] The Center for Research, Education, and Quality, MEDNAX Services/Pediatrix Medical Group/American Anesthesiology, 1301 Concord Terrace, Sunrise, FL 33323-2825, USA;
[b] School of Nursing, University of Pennsylvania, Philadelphia, PA, USA
* Corresponding author.
E-mail address: reese_clark@pediatrix.com

Clin Perinatol 41 (2014) 295–307
http://dx.doi.org/10.1016/j.clp.2014.02.001
0095-5108/14/$ – see front matter © 2014 Elsevier Inc. All rights reserved.
perinatology.theclinics.com

The evidence that poor intrauterine growth manifests as small for gestational age (SGA), excessive growth manifests as large for gestational age (LGA), and both influence health outcomes is not new[3–5] and remains a valuable consideration today.[6] Compared with premature infants born with normal weights for gestational age, SGA preterm infants have a higher mortality and are more likely to have postnatal growth failure, prolonged mechanical ventilation, and require treatment with postnatal steroids.[6] Being born SGA is associated with an increased risk of death or neurodevelopmental impairment. Similarly, infants born LGA are at increased risk for poor outcomes, including hypoglycemia, respiratory distress, obesity, and longer hospital stays.[7–10]

Although intrauterine growth restriction (IUGR) and SGA are commonly considered synonymous terms, the definitions and standards used to identify IUGR are different from those used to define SGA. A fetus with a diagnosis of IUGR may not meet the criteria for a diagnosis of SGA (usually defined as <10th percentile for age); however, both IUGR and SGA are associated with increased risk for poor health.[11–13]

How an infant grows after being born prematurely also is important. Numerous articles demonstrate that infants born prematurely are at high risk for poor extrauterine growth (weight, length, and head circumference) when compared with estimates of growth that would have occurred had the infants remained in utero.[14–17] Risk factors associated with poor extrauterine growth in prematurely born infants include immaturity (low gestational age), SGA status, male gender, need for assisted ventilation on the day of birth, a history of necrotizing enterocolitis, need for respiratory support at 28 days of age, and exposure to steroids during the hospital course.[15] Risk factors that influence growth also impact other outcomes and make it difficult to assess the independent impact of early growth on long-term outcomes. Ehrenkranz and colleagues,[18] however, showed that the pattern of growth of prematurely born infants exerts a significant, and possibly independent, effect on neurodevelopmental status and growth outcome at 18 to 22 months' corrected age. Data on how well individual sites promote normal growth show that some neonatal intensive care units (NICUs) perform better than other units.[19–21] Site performance can be improved, and one method for improving the growth of preterm infants admitted for intensive care is simply to monitor their growth and thereby diagnose and treat growth failure at an early stage.[21]

The concept that adequate nutritional status and normal growth are important is well accepted. How to assess the adequacy of nutrition and how to define appropriate growth remains an area of active debate. Our goal is to review how growth is assessed at birth and during the hospital stay of prematurely born infants, and to offer a standardized approach.

ASSESSMENT OF GROWTH STATUS AT BIRTH

In the NICU and the healthy newborn nursery, assessment of growth begins at birth. The assessments of weight, length, and head circumference are all equally important and must be a part of every admission examination. Meaningful assignment of SGA and LGA classification therefore requires the following: accurate knowledge of gestational age; accurate measurement at birth of weight, length, and head circumference; and cutoff values based on reference data from a relevant population,[22] all of which are a challenge to achieve. For example, estimated gestational age is often not precise and most experts would argue that gestational age precision is, at best, plus or minus 2 weeks. Although weights that use an electronic balance are quite accurate, individual head and length measurements may be less reliable in the clinical setting. Furthermore, the assessment tools (eg, growth curves) used to evaluate growth differ based on numerous factors, such as sample selection (eg, population sample of infants compared with "healthy" infants by excluding for infant/maternal factors that may affect infant growth/size), how gestational age is defined (eg, completed or mid-weeks),[22] combined or gender-specific curves,[23,24] and combined or race/ethnicity-specific curves.[25]

In the creation of growth curves, decisions related to these factors may change the cutoffs used to define "high risk" in the NICU. Both gender and race/ethnicity also confound the assignment of SGA and LGA.[24–27] The impact of assigning SGA and LGA independent of gender and race/ethnicity leads to errors in assignment.[24–26] Gender/ethnicity-specific birth-weight distributions are significantly better at identifying the infants at higher risk of neonatal morbidity.[25] Thus, understanding how an assessment tool was created can help clinicians decide which tool best suits their purpose and clinical setting. Assigning the precise percentile rank of any given growth measurement for an individual newborn at a particular postnatal age in a specific population requires data that are specific for race/ethnicity, gender, environment, maternal health, and population. For monitoring the pattern of growth, these factors are less important, because trends over time are more important than precise assessment of population-specific percentiles.

Normal gestation is longer than 37 weeks, and infants born "preterm" are, by definition, not normal. One reason infants are delivered prematurely is because they are not growing well (ie, IUGR).[28,29] The distributions of birth-growth parameters by estimated gestational age are not parametric (not normally distributed in a bell-shaped curve). Instead they are slightly skewed toward lower values (**Fig. 1**). Moreover, variables that alter growth are difficult to collect and may be missing from administrative data sets (eg, birth certificate data). Known influences on intrauterine growth are

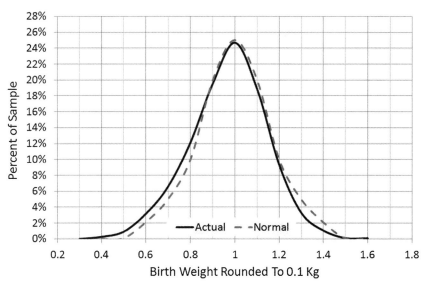

Fig. 1. A histogram plot of birth weight for inborn infants without anomalies that were reported to the Pediatrix Clinical Data Warehouse who had a gestational age of 27 weeks. The *solid line* is the observed distribution of birth weights and the *dashed line* is a normal/parametric distribution. Compared to a normal distribution, the observed distribution is shifted to the left demonstrating that preterm birth is associated with selection bias favoring lower weights than would be predicted. This finding is consistent with the clinical observation that one of the reasons preterm infants are delivered early is due to poor intrauterine growth.

maternal factors, such as smoking, hypertension, preeclampsia, diabetes, and repeated courses of antenatal steroids.[30] Without a prospective study, it is difficult to exclude infants who are exposed to perinatal risk factors for abnormal intrauterine growth, and the percentiles on any set of growth charts will be partly affected by how well patients with abnormal growth due to maternal illness/practices are excluded.[28,29] All of these confounding variables make it difficult to define precise growth assessment standards that are specific to the population being assessed. To enhance accuracy, we need more precise measurements based on "normal" population samples.

One potential approach would be to assign a percentile or z score to each growth parameter, rather than assigning a more general SGA or LGA classification. The tools for making these assignments based on recent growth curves are readily available and easily adaptable to electronic health records.[23,24,31] Birth weight, length, and head circumference are continuous values; the derivatives (percentile or z score) assigned to the measurement are also continuous values and can be considered as such. When a patient is assigned a designation of SGA or LGA, however, a continuous value is changed to a categorical value (for example <10th percentile for SGA and >90th percentile for LGA). Just as each 100-g increase in birth weight is associated with an increased likelihood that a prematurely born infant will survive,[32] infants with birth weights at the 60th percentile are more likely to survive than infants with birth weights at the 30th percentile.[32] Rather than making a categorical assignment, it is more helpful to assign a percentile or z score that provides a measure of how the newborn's growth measurements compare with a reference population by using a standardized growth curve. None of the available standardized growth curves are perfect, and continued research is needed to make them more clinically useful.[23] Clinicians should pick a single standard and validate that standard against the patient population they are assessing, similar that reported by Olsen and colleagues.[24]

Equally important is that *infants' potential for future growth is influenced by where they start at birth*. An infant born LGA tends to stay large for gestation as she or he grows in the NICU, and infants born SGA tend to stay SGA. The growth velocities may be similar if they are following their birth percentile. Crossing percentiles for any measurement (losing or gaining) suggest abnormal growth. For example, an infant with a head circumference at birth that is at the 50th percentile who leaves the NICU with a head circumference below the 10th percentile (poor head growth) is at serious risk for neurodevelopmental problems.[18] If the same infant has a head circumference above the 90th percentile at discharge, growth was not normal and hydrocephalus or other causes for abnormalities should be considered.

Assigning an infant a set of percentiles for weight, length, and head circumference at birth gives the clinician an estimate of risk for morbidity. It also allows the clinician to estimate the goals for growth based on weight, length, and head circumference targets for achieving the same percentile at discharge from the hospital. Failure to achieve normal growth targets is important in assessing health and future risk.[6,18]

MONITORING GROWTH IN THE NICU

The second reason for using growth charts is to monitor postnatal growth of prematurely born infants.

The Problem with Growth Velocity As a Singular Measure of Growth in the NICU

The use of growth velocity alone without the plotting of growth measurements on standardized growth charts is not an ideal way to assess adequate nutrition and adequate growth. Fetal growth is dynamic and not easily defined by a single slope (**Fig. 2**). Using size at birth as an estimate of fetal growth, fetal growth velocity can be calculated over each consecutive week and these calculations show that fetal growth changes with gestational age (**Tables 1** and **2**).[24] From estimates of fetal growth and observed growth of premature infants, targets for growth can be suggested: weight gain of 18 to 20 g/kg per day, length growth of 1.1 to 1.4 cm per week, and head circumference growth from 0.9 to 1.1 cm per week.[18,24] The problem with this approach is that it provides no frame of reference with respect to normal. Plotting growth on standardized growth charts gives a measure of both growth velocity and the deviation from fetal growth.[16–18]

After delivery, infants lose weight.[33] Healthy newborn infants regain their birth weight within the first 2 weeks. A similar pattern is seen in preterm infants. During the first 2 to 3 weeks following birth, growth is poor (**Fig. 3**). The most concerning observation is that this poor growth is not limited to weight gain alone but is also seen with length and head growth.[34–37] When assessing growth velocity, some investigators do not include this period of poor growth. Growth velocity is calculated for the period between the time that the infant regained birth weight and when that infant was discharged.[18] For the clinician providing daily care, the targets need to be based on data points that are closer together and based on what is safely achievable.

The Case for Using Standardized Growth Charts to Assess Adequacy of Growth

During well-child visits, children are plotted on growth charts that are based on cross-sectional studies; this assessment is an important measurement in health and well-being. Just as there are debates about which sets of charts are the best tools

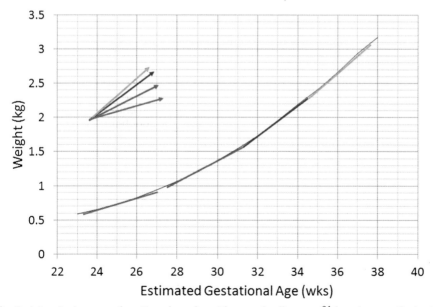

Fig. 2. Intrauterine growth pattern based on Olsen and colleagues'[24] female growth charts. Similar to **Table 1**, this chart shows how growth velocity changes with increasing gestational age. Growth velocity increases with increasing postnatal gestational age. Growth velocity changes with increasing postnatal gestational age. Growth velocity increases with increasing gestational age until term gestation, when it decelerates. Growth velocity changes: 23 to 27 weeks (purple); 27 to 31 weeks (red); 31 to 35 weeks (deep blue); 35 to 38 weeks (green).

Table 1
Estimated intrauterine weight gain velocity by EGA based on Olsen charts

	Female			Male		
	Median Weight (g)	Change (g/d)	Change (g/kg/d)	Median Weight (g)	Change (g/d)	Change (g/kg/d)
23	584			622		
24	651	9.6	16	689	9.6	15
25	737	12.3	19	777	12.6	18
26	827	12.9	18	888	15.9	20
27	936	15.6	19	1001	16.1	18
28	1061	17.9	19	1138	19.6	20
29	1204	20.4	19	1277	19.9	17
30	1373	24.1	20	1435	22.6	18
31	1546	24.7	18	1633	28.3	20
32	1731	26.4	17	1823	27.1	17
33	1956	32.1	19	2058	33.6	18
34	2187	33	17	2288	32.9	16
35	2413	32.3	15	2529	34.4	15
36	2664	35.9	15	2798	38.4	15
37	2937	39	15	3058	37.1	13
38	3173	33.7	11	3319	37.3	12
39	3338	23.6	7	3476	22.4	7
40	3454	16.6	5	3582	15.1	4

Abbreviation: EGA, estimated gestational age.

for monitoring growth from birth to adolescence, there are debates about how to best monitor postnatal growth in prematurely born infants.[23,31] Development of fetal growth charts based on observation of a healthy cohort of women who deliver a healthy infant at term would be ideal; this work is ongoing (http://intergrowth21.org.uk/). Unfortunately, although intrauterine growth charts based on ultrasound-estimated fetal size might be more representative of "normal" fetal growth,[28] and reflect the growth of the infants delivered at term, determination of an estimated weight of a fetus during pregnancy is limited by the ability to accurately obtain the measurements.[38] This approach becomes even more difficult when developing charts for head circumference and length.

Poor growth, termed extrauterine growth restriction, is common in the NICU. Growth charts allow the clinician to monitor how far a given infant is falling behind and to adjust the nutritional approach accordingly (**Fig. 4**). The health benefits of human milk are well recognized; however, the precise nutritional content of fresh human milk is variable and often not measured. Monitoring growth allows clinicians to intervene in preterm infants who are falling behind or whose growth status is decreasing from birth percentiles. In this setting, the precise percentile measurement is less important than the pattern of growth over time. Weight is measured daily and can be easily plotted in electronic medical records. The assessment of head circumference and length are more commonly done once a week. These assessments are as important as any laboratory value or procedural evaluation. Without visualizing the pattern of growth, diagnosis and treatment of growth failure is delayed and long-term outcome may be altered.[17,18] Although poor weight gain appears to be

Table 2
Estimated intrauterine weekly length and head circumferences growth velocity by EGA based on Olsen charts

	Female				Male			
	Median Length (cm)	Change (cm/wk)	Median Head Circumference (cm)	Change (cm/wk)	Median Length (cm)	Change (cm/wk)	Median Head Circumference (cm)	Change (cm/wk)
23	29.9		20.9		30.3		21.3	
24	31.1	1.2	21.8	0.9	31.5	1.2	22.2	0.9
25	32.3	1.2	22.7	0.9	32.9	1.4	23.2	1
26	33.6	1.3	23.6	0.9	34.3	1.4	24.2	1
27	35	1.4	24.5	0.9	35.7	1.4	25.2	1
28	36.5	1.5	25.5	1	37.2	1.5	26.1	0.9
29	38	1.5	26.5	1	38.7	1.5	27.1	1
30	39.5	1.5	27.5	1	40.1	1.4	28	0.9
31	41	1.5	28.4	0.9	41.6	1.5	28.9	0.9
32	42.3	1.3	29.3	0.9	43	1.4	29.9	1
33	43.7	1.4	30.2	0.9	44.4	1.4	30.8	0.9
34	45	1.3	31.1	0.9	45.7	1.3	31.6	0.8
35	46.2	1.2	31.9	0.8	46.9	1.2	32.4	0.8
36	47.4	1.2	32.7	0.8	48.1	1.2	33.2	0.8
37	48.5	1.1	33.3	0.6	49.3	1.2	33.9	0.7
38	49.5	1	33.7	0.4	50.2	0.9	34.4	0.5
39	50.2	0.7	34	0.3	51	0.8	34.6	0.2
40	50.8	0.6	34.3	0.3	51.6	0.6	34.8	0.2

Abbreviation: EGA, estimated gestational age.

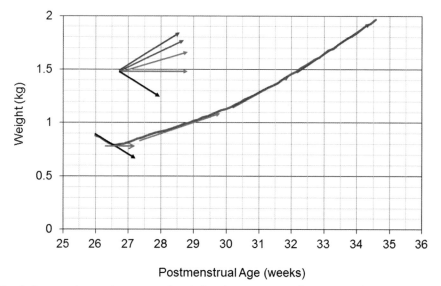

Fig. 3. Postnatal growth pattern of an infant born at 26 weeks' estimated gestational age based on observation made in 1000 inborn infants who survived to be discharged. Note that growth velocity continues to accelerate through term gestation. Growth velocity changes following birth for an infant born at 26 weeks estimated gestational age: 0 to 5 days (black); 5 to 10 days (light blue); 10 to 28 days (light grey); 28 to 42 days (deep blue); 42 to 56 days (brown). (*Data from* the Pediatrix Clinical Data Warehouse 2009–2010.)

SINGLETON HOSPITAL
STAFF LIBRARY

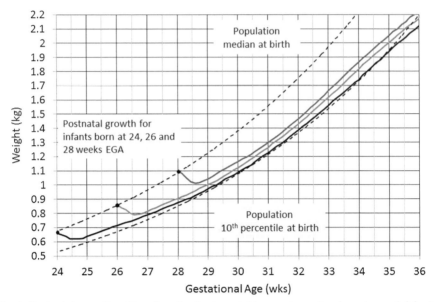

Fig. 4. Postnatal growth pattern (median body weight vs postmenstrual age in weeks) for infants born at 24, 26, and 28 weeks' estimated gestational age based on observations made in inborn infants who survived to be discharged. The reference is based on the population-based 10th and 50th percentiles and the data are from the Pediatrix Clinical Data Warehouse. For each group of infants, the median weights fall away from the intrauterine growth charts, so that by 36 weeks, the median postnatal weight for each group of preterm infants is approaching the 10th percentile for the estimated fetal weight of a similar group of infants who did not deliver prematurely. Similar to Ehrenkranz and colleagues,[16] the birth weights of each group of infants are similar to the birth weights of the infants shown on the reference intrauterine growth chart (they start at the 50th percentile). As they grow in the NICU, most of the infants born between 24 and 28 weeks' gestation do not achieve the median birth weight of the reference fetus of the same postmenstrual age, and many are discharged with a weight less than the 10th percentile.

the most predictive of poor outcome, all 3 measurements of growth (weight, length, and head circumference) are valuable and essential to understanding proportional growth.

Which Intrauterine Growth Charts Should Be Used As a Reference

Two sets of charts are commonly used in the NICU.[23,24] Between 23 and 37 weeks, both the gender-specific Fenton and Olsen charts are similar.[23] There are 2 important distinctions between these 2 sets of charts. First, the reformatted Olsen charts that include the World Health Organization (WHO) charts, interface the Olsen and WHO charts at 39 weeks' postmenstrual age (instead of 40 weeks), because 39 weeks is the median age for the WHO definition of full-term (range 37–41 weeks) and 39 weeks is the median age of US births (http://wonder.cdc.gov/controller/datarequest/D66). Second, the Olsen charts and WHO charts are each based on independent sets of data and for that reason are not connected. The smoothing process that joins the 2 distinctive charts distorts the estimates of percentile lines for both charts.

Although the median hospital stay of prematurely born infants is 36 to 37 weeks' postmenstrual age and most infants do not need charts that go beyond 37 weeks, critically ill preterm infants often require longer hospitalizations and therefore need to be transitioned from a "fetal" reference chart to an infant chart. The WHO charts are considered the standards for monitoring growth of children from birth into childhood (0–24 months).[2,39] To monitor growth in preterm infants as they grow beyond 37 weeks requires the addition of the WHO charts to intrauterine growth charts. The pattern of preterm infant growth is consistent with intrauterine growth between 23 and 37 weeks and the deceleration in growth velocity seen in growth as the fetus approaches 40 weeks' gestational age (see **Tables 1** and **2**) is not seen in the healthy preterm infant growing well in the NICU.[31] The reformatted Olsen charts are available at (http://www.pediatrix.com/workfiles/NICUGrowthCurves7.30.pdf). The Fenton charts are available at http://www.ucalgary.ca/fenton/2013chart.

We believe it is less important which set of charts is used than it is to routinely plot growth over time to look for accelerations and decelerations. There is general agreement that gender-specific charts should be used when assessing percentiles. What is less certain is whether we need population-specific charts based on country or race/ethnicity. Again, assessing the precise percentile of any given growth measurement at any specific postnatal age, population-specific data are important, but for monitoring the pattern of growth the data are less important.

MONITORING THE PROPORTIONALITY OF WEIGHT GROWTH RELATIVE TO STATURE

Body mass index (BMI) is an anthropometric index of weight relative to stature, defined as body weight in kilograms divided by length in meters squared. BMI is considered a reliable indicator of body fatness for most children and teens.[40] There is no routinely used measure of body proportionality, like BMI, to assess body size and associated risk in preterm infants in the NICU setting. An elevated BMI in children and adults is correlated with higher body fat composition[41,42] and risk of later related diseases.[43–46] Thus, BMI is an important part of the clinical assessment for these age groups. In preterm infants, rapid postnatal growth, fat accumulation, and the association of these factors with adverse outcomes[47–55] has increased interest in the composition of postnatal growth of preterm infants.[56,57] Because body composition is not routinely measured in the NICU, a proxy such as BMI may be a useful clinical tool for preterm infants.

Historically, the growth assessment of preterm infants has focused on rates of growth velocity and growth status based on size-for-age. This method evaluates how an infant is growing compared with fetuses of the same age, as recommended, yet it does not identify growth that is *disproportionate* or weight gain that might be too low or too high for an infant's length. A rough estimate of appropriate weight gain relative to length gain (or *body proportionality*) can be made by comparing weight-for-age and length-for-age percentiles, determined by plotting these on intrauterine growth charts. However, a measure of body proportionality provides a simple and possibly more accurate method of identifying, quantifying, and tracking disproportionate growth by comparing weight relative to length in one parameter.

A study of young preterm infants evaluated the utility of Lubchenco and colleagues' *weight-for-length* (defined as ponderal index or weight/length[3]-for-age[5]) curve in the NICU and found that it categorized infants as small, appropriate, and large in a manner different from the weight-for-age curve.[14] Most of the infants who were categorized as small weight-for-age (or SGA) were categorized as appropriate weight-for-length at birth and discharge (77% and 81%); 19% of the infants were categorized as appropriate weight-for-age (AGA) at discharge but were large weight-for-length. The measure of body proportionality provided different information about weight growth status in preterm infants than weight-for-age alone.[14] Others also have described variation in growth status when assessed by weight-for-age versus body fat or its proxies (ie, measures of body proportionality).[54,58] Similar to other periods of the life cycle, a combination of these measures should help clinicians to make more informed and individualized nutrition-care decisions that have the potential to improve outcomes.

The ideal measure of body proportionality for preterm infants of all gestational ages, however, lacks agreement.[54] Weight-for-length ratios are good candidates, as these measurements are routinely performed in the clinical setting. The current utility of the Lubchenco ponderal index curve is limited because of its lack of generalizability to contemporary US NICUs and it may not accurately capture the weight-for-length relationship of preterm infants for all gestational ages.[59] Using the methods of Benn,[60] who defined the "ideal" weight-for-length ratio as that most highly correlated with weight and least correlated with length/height, Cole and colleagues[59] found that the ideal ratio for infants born between 33 and 39 weeks' gestation was the ponderal index, BMI for infants born after 39 weeks. Infants born before 33 weeks' gestation were not studied.

Despite the benefits of including a measure of body proportionality in the growth assessment of preterm infants, it has several important limitations. First, BMI is designed to identify and quantify disproportionality between weight and length (ie, asymmetrical growth). As a result, symmetric growth restriction or excess that results in stunted weight and length or excessive weight and length, respectively, will not be identified by a BMI or other measures of body proportionality. The second limitation of BMI is that it does not distinguish between body fat mass and fat-free mass; thus, a high BMI (indicating overweight-for-length) could be due to an excess of body fat mass or a deficiency of fat-free mass. When the body composition of former preterm infants at corrected full-term age is compared with that of full-term infants, fat mass is equivalent or greater and fat-free mass is less in former preterm infants, resulting in higher percentage of body fat estimates.[34,56,57,61] As more body composition data for preterm infants become available, the relationships between measures of body proportionality and body composition and outcomes will need to be thoroughly explored.[54]

SUMMARY

The assessment of intrauterine and extrauterine growth in preterm infants is an essential component of high-quality neonatal care. New and better tools for assessing growth are available and represent important steps forward in the provision of maternal/fetal and neonatal intensive care. How a fetus and how a prematurely born infant grow influence outcome, and failure to diagnose and treat growth problems can lead to poor outcomes. What represents healthy growth and decreasing the variability between growth outcomes among NICUs are essential areas for future research.

REFERENCES

1. Promoting optimal monitoring of child growth in Canada: using the new World Health Organization growth charts—executive summary. Paediatr Child Health 2010;15:77–83.
2. Grummer-Strawn LM, Reinold C, Krebs NF. Use of World Health Organization and CDC growth charts for children aged 0-59 months in the United States. MMWR Recomm Rep 2010;59:1–15.

3. Lubchenco LO. Classification of high risk infants by birth weight and gestational age: an overview. Major Probl Clin Pediatr 1976;14:1–279.
4. Lubchenco LO, Searls DT, Brazie JV. Neonatal mortality rate: relationship to birth weight and gestational age. J Pediatr 1972;81:814–22.
5. Lubchenco LO, Hansman C, Boyd E. Intrauterine growth in length and head circumference as estimated from live births at gestational ages from 26 to 42 weeks. Pediatrics 1966;37:403–8.
6. De Jesus LC, Pappas A, Shankaran S, et al. Outcomes of small for gestational age infants born at <27 weeks' gestation. J Pediatr 2013;163:55–60.
7. Morgan K, Rahman M, Atkinson M, et al. Association of diabetes in pregnancy with child weight at birth, age 12 months and 5 years—a population-based electronic cohort study. PLoS One 2013;8:e79803.
8. Boney CM, Verma A, Tucker R, et al. Metabolic syndrome in childhood: association with birth weight, maternal obesity, and gestational diabetes mellitus. Pediatrics 2005;115:e290–6.
9. Weissmann-Brenner A, Simchen MJ, Zilberberg E, et al. Maternal and neonatal outcomes of large for gestational age pregnancies. Acta Obstet Gynecol Scand 2012;91:844–9.
10. Pasupathy D, McCowan LM, Poston L, et al. Perinatal outcomes in large infants using customised birthweight centiles and conventional measures of high birthweight. Paediatr Perinat Epidemiol 2012;26:543–52.
11. Barker DJ, Forsen T, Eriksson JG, et al. Growth and living conditions in childhood and hypertension in adult life: a longitudinal study. J Hypertens 2002;20:1951–6.
12. Zaw W, Gagnon R, da Silva O. The risks of adverse neonatal outcome among preterm small for gestational age infants according to neonatal versus fetal growth standards. Pediatrics 2003;111:1273–7.
13. Garite TJ, Clark R, Thorp JA. Intrauterine growth restriction increases morbidity and mortality among premature neonates. Am J Obstet Gynecol 2004;191:481–7.
14. Olsen IE, Lawson ML, Meinzen-Derr J, et al. Use of a body proportionality index for growth assessment of preterm infants. J Pediatr 2009;154:486–91.
15. Clark RH, Thomas P, Peabody J. Extrauterine growth restriction remains a serious problem in prematurely born neonates. Pediatrics 2003;111:986–90.
16. Ehrenkranz RA, Younes N, Lemons JA, et al. Longitudinal growth of hospitalized very low birth weight infants. Pediatrics 1999;104:280–9.
17. Ehrenkranz RA. Extrauterine growth restriction: is it preventable? J Pediatr (Rio J) 2014;90(1):1–3.
18. Ehrenkranz RA, Dusick AM, Vohr BR, et al. Growth in the neonatal intensive care unit influences neurodevelopmental and growth outcomes of extremely low birth weight infants. Pediatrics 2006;117:1253–61.
19. Blackwell MT, Eichenwald EC, McAlmon K, et al. Interneonatal intensive care unit variation in growth rates and feeding practices in healthy moderately premature infants. J Perinatol 2005;25:478–85.
20. Olsen IE, Richardson DK, Schmid CH, et al. Intersite differences in weight growth velocity of extremely premature infants. Pediatrics 2002;110:1125–32.
21. Bloom BT, Mulligan J, Arnold C, et al. Improving growth of very low birth weight infants in the first 28 days. Pediatrics 2003;112:8–14.
22. Rochow N, Raja P, Straube S, et al. Misclassification of newborns due to systematic error in plotting birth weight percentile values. Pediatrics 2012;130:e347–51.

23. Fenton TR, Kim JH. A systematic review and meta-analysis to revise the Fenton growth chart for preterm infants. BMC Pediatr 2013;13:59.

24. Olsen IE, Groveman SA, Lawson ML, et al. New intrauterine growth curves based on United States data. Pediatrics 2010;125:e214–24.

25. Hanley GE, Janssen PA. Ethnicity-specific birthweight distributions improve identification of term newborns at risk for short-term morbidity. Am J Obstet Gynecol 2013;209:428.e1–6.

26. Thomas P, Peabody J, Turnier V, et al. A new look at intrauterine growth and the impact of race, altitude, and gender. Pediatrics 2000;106:E21.

27. Alexander GR, Kogan M, Bader D, et al. US birth weight/gestational age-specific neonatal mortality: 1995-1997 rates for whites, Hispanics, and blacks. Pediatrics 2003;111:e61–6.

28. Cooke RW. Conventional birth weight standards obscure fetal growth restriction in preterm infants. Arch Dis Child Fetal Neonatal Ed 2007;92:F189–92.

29. Salomon LJ, Bernard JP, Ville Y. Estimation of fetal weight: reference range at 20-36 weeks' gestation and comparison with actual birth-weight reference range. Ultrasound Obstet Gynecol 2007;29:550–5.

30. Lausman A, Kingdom J, Gagnon R, et al. Intrauterine growth restriction: screening, diagnosis, and management. J Obstet Gynaecol Can 2013;35:741–57.

31. Fenton TR, Nasser R, Eliasziw M, et al. Validating the weight gain of preterm infants between the reference growth curve of the fetus and the term infant. BMC Pediatr 2013;13:92.

32. Tyson JE, Parikh NA, Langer J, et al. Intensive care for extreme prematurity—moving beyond gestational age. N Engl J Med 2008;358:1672–81.

33. Noel-Weiss J, Courant G, Woodend AK. Physiological weight loss in the breastfed neonate: a systematic review. Open Med 2008;2:e99–110.

34. Ramel SE, Demerath EW, Gray HL, et al. The relationship of poor linear growth velocity with neonatal illness and two-year neurodevelopment in preterm infants. Neonatology 2012;102:19–24.

35. Berngard SC, Berngard JB, Krebs NF, et al. Newborn length predicts early infant linear growth retardation and disproportionately high weight gain in a low-income population. Early Hum Dev 2013;89:967–72.

36. Miller J, Makrides M, Gibson RA, et al. Effect of increasing protein content of human milk fortifier on growth in preterm infants born at <31 wk gestation: a randomized controlled trial. Am J Clin Nutr 2012;95:648–55.

37. Olsen IE, Harris CL, Lawson L, et al. Higher protein intake improves length, not weight, z-scores in preterm infants. J Pediatr Gastroenterol Nutr 2013 [Epub ahead of print]. PubMed PMID: 24231639.

38. Ehrenkranz RA. Estimated fetal weights versus birth weights: should the reference intrauterine growth curves based on birth weights be retired? Arch Dis Child Fetal Neonatal Ed 2007;92:F161–2.

39. de OM, Onyango AW, Borghi E, et al. Comparison of the World Health Organization (WHO) child growth standards and the National Center for Health Statistics/WHO international growth reference: implications for child health programmes. Public Health Nutr 2006;9:942–7.

40. Mei Z, Grummer-Strawn LM, Pietrobelli A, et al. Validity of body mass index compared with other body-composition screening indexes for the assessment of body fatness in children and adolescents. Am J Clin Nutr 2002;75:978–85.

41. Ellis KJ. Selected body composition methods can be used in field studies. J Nutr 2001;131:1589S–95S.

42. Gallagher D, Visser M, Sepulveda D, et al. How useful is body mass index for comparison of body fatness across age, sex, and ethnic groups? Am J Epidemiol 1996;143:228–39.

43. Dabelea D, Harrod CS. Role of developmental overnutrition in pediatric obesity and type 2 diabetes. Nutr Rev 2013;71(Suppl 1):S62–7.

44. Park MH, Falconer C, Viner RM, et al. The impact of childhood obesity on morbidity and mortality in adulthood: a systematic review. Obes Rev 2012;13:985–1000.

45. Li L, Pinot de MA, Power C. Predicting cardiovascular disease risk factors in midadulthood from childhood body mass index: utility of different cutoffs for childhood body mass index. Am J Clin Nutr 2011;93:1204–11.

46. Juonala M, Magnussen CG, Berenson GS, et al. Childhood adiposity, adult adiposity, and cardiovascular risk factors. N Engl J Med 2011;365:1876–85.

47. Druet C, Stettler N, Sharp S, et al. Prediction of childhood obesity by infancy weight gain: an individual-level meta-analysis. Paediatr Perinat Epidemiol 2012;26:19–26.

48. Durmus B, Mook-Kanamori DO, Holzhauer S, et al. Growth in foetal life and infancy is associated with abdominal adiposity at the age of 2 years: the generation R study. Clin Endocrinol (Oxf) 2010;72:633–40.

49. Ong KK. Catch-up growth in small for gestational age babies: good or bad? Curr Opin Endocrinol Diabetes Obes 2007;14:30–4.

50. Ong KK, Loos RJ. Rapid infancy weight gain and subsequent obesity: systematic reviews and hopeful suggestions. Acta Paediatr 2006;95:904–8.

51. Euser AM, Finken MJ, Keijzer-Veen MG, et al. Associations between prenatal and infancy weight gain and BMI, fat mass, and fat distribution in young adulthood: a prospective cohort study in males and females born very preterm. Am J Clin Nutr 2005;81:480–7.

52. Johnson MJ, Wootton SA, Leaf AA, et al. Preterm birth and body composition at term equivalent age: a systematic review and meta-analysis. Pediatrics 2012; 130:e640–9.

53. Ramel SE, Gray HL, Ode KL, et al. Body composition changes in preterm infants following hospital discharge: comparison with term infants. J Pediatr Gastroenterol Nutr 2011;53:333–8.

54. Holston A, Stokes T, Olsen C, et al. Novel noninvasive anthropometric measure in preterm and full-term infants: normative values for waist circumference: length ratio at birth. Pediatr Res 2013;74:299–306.

55. Stokes TA, Holston A, Olsen C, et al. Preterm infants of lower gestational age at birth have greater waist circumference-length ratio and ponderal index at term age than preterm infants of higher gestational ages. J Pediatr 2012;161:735–41.

56. Griffin IJ, Cooke RJ. Development of whole body adiposity in preterm infants. Early Hum Dev 2012;88(Suppl 1):S19–24.

57. Cooke RJ, Griffin I. Altered body composition in preterm infants at hospital discharge. Acta Paediatr 2009;98:1269–73.

58. Schmelzle HR, Quang DN, Fusch G, et al. Birth weight categorization according to gestational age does not reflect percentage body fat in term and preterm newborns. Eur J Pediatr 2007;166:161–7.

59. Cole TJ, Henson GL, Tremble JM, et al. Birthweight for length: ponderal index, body mass index or Benn index? Ann Hum Biol 1997;24:289–98.

60. Benn RT. Some mathematical properties of weight-for-height indices used as measures of adiposity. Br J Prev Soc Med 1971;25:42–50.

61. Simon L, Borrego P, Darmaun D, et al. Effect of sex and gestational age on neonatal body composition. Br J Nutr 2013;109:1105–8.

Linear Growth and Neurodevelopmental Outcomes

Katie M. Pfister, MD, Sara E. Ramel, MD*

KEYWORDS

- Linear growth • Fat-free mass • Inflammation • Outcomes • Neurodevelopment
- Premature infants • Very low birth weight

KEY POINTS

- Premature infants exhibit disproportionate growth characterized by reduced length/height and fat-free mass (FFM), as well as neurodevelopmental delay.
- Growth should no longer be defined as weight gain alone, as increases or stunting in other metrics are associated with lasting effects on neurodevelopment.
- Brain maturation is characterized by critical periods of growth, each with specific nutrient needs.
- Protein status plays an important role in FFM accretion, neurogenesis, and neuronal differentiation.
- Early inflammation and illness have a long-term negative influence on linear growth and in FFM gains, as well as on later neurodevelopment.

INTRODUCTION

Despite recent improvements in nutritional support, premature infants continue to exhibit disproportionate growth (characterized by reduced length/height and fat-free mass [FFM], and increased relative adiposity), as well as neurodevelopmental delay. Recent literature suggests that some of the same factors (eg, nutritional and inflammatory) are responsible for both outcomes, by directly and negatively affecting both developing neurons and white matter, and suppressing the growth hormone (GH)/insulin-like growth factor 1 (IGF-1) axes. Reduced FFM accretion and linear growth are associated with a risk to the developing brain. To date, neonatal nutritional strategies have been ineffective in preventing failure of linear growth and its attendant risk to cognitive development, in part because of a lack of thorough understanding of what

The authors have no disclosures.

Division of Neonatology, Department of Pediatrics, University of Minnesota, 2450 Riverside Avenue East Building MB 630, Minneapolis, MN 55454, USA

* Corresponding author.

E-mail address: sramel@umn.edu

0095-5108/14/$ – see front matter © 2014 Elsevier Inc. All rights reserved.

causes suppression of linear growth and in part because of an inappropriate emphasis on defining "growth" as weight gain. A potential change in care to improve developmental outcomes might include more careful monitoring of linear growth and body composition (including FFM), accompanied by strategic nutritional and nonnutritional interventions aimed at supporting FFM growth. The latter could include strategies to reduce the duration of illness and the number of inflammatory events.

INCIDENCE OF GROWTH FAILURE IN PREMATURE INFANTS

In 2011, the rate of preterm birth in the United States remained greater than 11%.[1] According to a review from the National Institute of Child Health and Human Development, the rate of growth failure among VLBW preterm infants remains unacceptably high, with 79% weighing less than the 10th percentile at 36 weeks.[2] Hack and colleagues[3] reported that many of these infants remain underweight and short for age (<2 standard deviations [SD]) at 20 months corrected age for prematurity, and that very low birth weight (VLBW) males remain small and short into adulthood.

The prevalence and importance of poor weight gain in preterm infants has been widely cited for decades. Although first described in 1981,[4] the incidence, persistence, and significance of linear-growth failure has only recently reemerged as a topic of importance. This renewed emphasis is particularly important because linear growth and gains in FFM closely index organ growth, and specifically the brain, in other populations. Multiple recently published studies have described prolonged suppression of linear growth in preterm infants beyond 18 to 24 months corrected age for prematurity (**Fig. 1**).[5–7]

In each of these studies, length z-scores were more severely depressed and remained lower longer than z-scores of weight and head circumference[6,7] and body mass index (kg/m^2).[5,6] This finding is unlike the classic undernutrition anthropometric pattern of growth failure whereby weight is compromised but length and head circumference are spared. The body habitus of excessively suppressed linear growth (ie, the

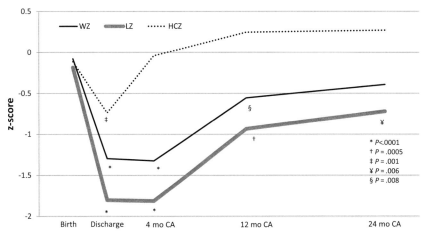

Fig. 1. Growth of very low birth weight preterm infants from birth to 24 months corrected age illustrating persistent linear stunting. P values refer to statistical significance of the difference between the mean growth z-score at each time point compared with the mean z-score at birth. HCZ, head circumference z-score; LZ, length z-score; WZ, weight z-score. (*From* Ramel SE, Demerath EW, Gray HL, et al. The relationship of poor linear growth velocity with neonatal illness and 2 year neurodevelopment in preterm infants. Neonatology 2012;102:21; with permission.)

"short, fat baby") suggests that nonnutritional factors may also play a role in this suppression.

Linear growth reflects FFM accretion. However, accurate linear growth measurements can be difficult to obtain. With the recent addition of infant air-displacement plethysmography, repeat noninvasive body composition measurements in infants, including those born prematurely, has become more feasible, and a plethora of research data monitoring body composition has become available. Not unexpectedly, it has been recently noted that preterm infants also have less FFM than term born infants when measured at term corrected age.[8,9] Two small studies have documented that this difference has subsided by 3 to 4 months corrected age[9,10]; however, further long-term studies on body composition are needed.

DEFINITIONS OF GROWTH

Growth of the preterm infant has historically been defined as weight gain over time. As weight gain and nutrition have been more extensively studied and their relationships with neurodevelopmental outcomes have been established, other growth parameters' relationships to outcome have also been assessed. Weight gain, head circumference, and linear growth all correlate with long-term outcomes in preterm infants. More recent studies have looked at body composition, quality of weight gain, and relationship to neurodevelopment as a more comprehensive evaluation of neonatal growth than any single anthropometric measurement alone. The American Academy of Pediatrics (AAP) recommends that the preterm infant achieve a growth rate similar to that of the intrauterine fetus of the same gestational age.[11] Although this recommendation continues to be interpreted as weight-gain velocity, growth in other metrics index important physiologic processes, including neurodevelopment.

Weight

Weight gain is the traditional metric of growth in the neonate. Weight represents the balance between energy intake and expenditure. The current recommendation for weight-gain velocity in the preterm infant is 15 to 18 g/kg/d, which approximates the weight gain of the fetus during the second through third trimester. However, higher velocities (20–30 g/kg/d) may be needed for extremely low birth weight infants to regain birth z-scores by term,[12] likely because of the need for catch-up growth after nutritional deficits in the first weeks of life. Although weight gain is associated with neurodevelopmental outcomes[13,14] and there are distinct recommendations for rates of weight gain in preterm neonates, this metric alone does not give a complete picture of the overall nutritional state of the infant, and can be confounded by nonnutritional weight gain (eg, edema).

Head Circumference

During the third trimester, the brain is undergoing tremendous changes characterized by increasing dendritic complexity and synaptic connectivity, which are reflected by increases in brain volume and surface area. In the absence of hydrocephalus, head circumference indexes the brain's growth and correlates with brain volume both post mortem and on magnetic resonance imaging (MRI).[15,16] The growth velocity of head circumference that mimics the fetus during the third trimester, and thus goal for growth of the preterm infant, is approximately 1 cm/week.[17] MRI findings in preterm infants who develop microcephaly by term corrected age show significant losses in deep nuclear gray matter (indicating neuronal loss, architecture, or both) compared with infants with normal z-scores.[16] Slow head growth has also been independently associated with delayed cortical gray matter maturation in preterm infants.[18] Stunting of head growth in both the neonatal[6,13,16,19] and postdischarge[19] periods is associated with poorer neurodevelopmental outcomes. However, microcephaly reflects severe malnutrition, owing to the head-sparing phenomenon, and thus loses its predictive value for neurodevelopment in most preterm infants who remain normocephalic during their hospital stay.

Length

Linear growth represents lean body mass and protein accretion[20,21] and also indexes organ growth and development, including the brain.[22] The AAP recommends that preterm infants grow similarly to the fetus,[11] but this guideline has been mostly applied to weight gain. As already described, the ideal weight gain to optimize neurodevelopmental outcomes has been studied extensively. However, ideal linear growth has yet to be defined. Intrauterine linear-growth velocity is approximately 1 cm/wk,[23] and therefore is the goal that most neonatologists currently follow. Given the increasing evidence that linear-growth suppression is associated with poorer cognitive outcomes,[5,7] length may be an important anthropometric biomarker for later neurodevelopment. Research is needed to determine optimal goals of linear growth for preterm infants so as to optimize later growth and neurodevelopmental outcomes.

Lower calorie and protein intakes during hospitalization are associated with prolonged suppression of linear growth.[7,24] In addition, inflammation, which increases protein breakdown, is associated with reduced length z-scores out to 24 months corrected age in preterm infants.[7] Strategies aimed at optimizing protein delivery with adequate energy support and reducing inflammation to decrease protein breakdown are 2 strategies that could potentially improve neurodevelopmental outcomes in this vulnerable population.

Body Composition

Body composition, the assessment of fat mass and FFM, has recently begun to be more thoroughly assessed in the preterm neonate. Like linear growth, FFM indexes organ growth and protein status. Improved FFM accretion has also recently been associated with improved speed of processing in preterm infants.[25] Fat also makes up a significant portion of the brain's structure. Fetal fat deposition begins during the third trimester, and in the fetus the percentage of body fat rapidly increases to roughly 15% of body weight by term.[26] Preterm infants, who are growing in the neonatal intensive care unit (NICU) during the corresponding postconceptional time period, have increased adiposity and less FFM at term corrected age when compared with their term gestation counterparts.[9,27,28] Moreover, fat stores in preterm infants are abnormally distributed, with decreased subcutaneous and increased intra-abdominal adipose tissue at term corrected age.[29] These alterations likely result from both nutritional abnormalities and maladaptive metabolism,[27,30,31] and the ideal body composition and how to achieve it in this population has not yet been defined. Given the concerns of increased adiposity and long-term metabolic risk in preterm infants, further research is needed to determine the ideal nutritional regimen for this population, and likely will require individualization to optimize growth, metabolic, and neurodevelopmental outcomes.

NUTRIENTS THAT AFFECT LINEAR GROWTH, FFM ACCRETION, AND NEURODEVELOPMENT

Although all nutrients are important for growth and brain development, certain nutrients are of particular significance in the developing preterm brain during critical periods of development. Nutrient deficiencies will have different effects based on when the deficit occurs and how the brain is using it at that time.[32] Deficits affect both the microstructure and the function of the brain. While a great deal is known about the effect of deficit or oversupplementation of certain nutrients in term infants and toddlers, many nutrients remain understudied, particularly in preterm infants. This population develops nutritional deficits during a period of tremendous neurologic change including increases in neuronal differentiation, dendritic complexity, synaptogenesis, and myelination. This article will focus specifically on those nutrients that are known to directly influence linear growth, FFM accretion, and neurodevelopment.

During the first few days to weeks of life, VLBW preterm infants accrue nutritional deficits that have been shown to influence long-term growth and neurodevelopment. This accrual is largely due to these infants' dependence on parenteral nutrition, and hesitancy to begin early enteral nutrition for fear of intolerance and development of necrotizing enterocolitis. Protein, in particular, has been limited owing to concerns over protein toxicity, stemming from previous trials that revealed metabolic acidosis, uremia, poor growth, and poorer neurodevelopmental outcomes in protein-supplemented infants.[33] However, current nutritional strategies use higher-quality protein at lower levels than previously reported, and have documented not only safety and tolerance of supplementation but also improved outcomes.[24,34–36]

Several recent studies, including a few clinical trials of protein supplementation (range of 4.2–4.8 g/kg/d), have shown improved linear growth and FFM accretion during hospitalization.[9,24,37,38] These findings are lasting in that infants receiving more aggressive protein supplementation while in the NICU continue to have higher amounts of FFM and improved length after discharge.[9,24,37]

Protein plays an important role in the developing brain, and is necessary for normal neurogenesis, dendritic arborization, synaptogenesis, and myelin production, as well as for cell signaling in the form of growth factors and neurotransmitters.[39] Between 26 weeks' gestation and term, the fetal brain transforms from a smooth, bilobed, 105-g organ to a complexly sulcated organ of 3.5 times this weight by term. The third trimester is a period of tremendous microscopic changes (see earlier discussion). Axonal and dendritic growth accounts for the large volume increase in the brain during the last trimester. This rapid pace of development leaves the preterm brain particularly vulnerable to the lack of critical nutrients that support this process, especially protein. Recent studies have consistently shown improved neurodevelopment in infants receiving more aggressive protein supplementation during hospitalization,[24,25,36,37] and these findings are lasting. Isaacs and colleagues[36] have documented improved brain volume and cognitive scores during adolescence in those infants receiving improved early protein intake.

Preterm infants have specific reductions in brain volume representing regional vulnerabilities (most significantly in the sensorimotor cortex but also including surrounding areas, corpus callosum, basal ganglia, amygdala, and hippocampus), which correspond with poorer cognitive outcome.[40] Even among "healthy" preterm infants and early term infants, shorter gestation is associated with decreases in gray-matter density at school age.[41] Reduction in gray matter is largely a function of reduced neuronal number and less neuronal complexity, both of which are induced by suboptimal protein intake. This process is likely controlled by cell-signaling pathways such as the mammalian target of rapamycin, which depends highly on branch-chain amino acids, IGF-1, and protein sufficiency, and is involved in neurogenesis, neuronal differentiation, and apoptosis.[42]

Protein also plays a role in stimulating neural growth factors such as IGF-1 and brain-derived neurotropic factor (BDNF). Animal studies have shown that protein restriction decreases serum and brain-tissue levels of IGF-1.[43,44] As associations between improved IGF-1 levels and lower risk of abnormal cognition in preterm infants[45] have recently been reported, the GH/IGF-1 axis may contribute to the association between improved protein status/linear growth and improved cognition.

Given the existing evidence, protein should be provided urgently to preterm infants. This administration should begin immediately after birth at approximately 3 g/kg/d via parenteral nutrition and be increased quickly to 4 to 4.5 g/kg/d. Protein supplementation should continue via human milk fortification and additional supplementation, as needed, to maintain these levels until at least hospital discharge. Infants receiving increased protein amounts (>3 g/kg/d) after discharge continue to have improved FFM accretion.[27] As associations with linear growth/FFM accretion and neurodevelopmental outcomes extend beyond hospital discharge, postdischarge fortification/protein supplementation should also be considered.

Although protein is a main driver of linear growth and organ development, other nutrients such as carbohydrates, fats, and zinc are also important, and their deficiencies can cause failure of linear growth despite optimal protein intake. Energy intake in the form of carbohydrates and fat is essential for adequate weight gain. Improved caloric intake has been shown to improve neurodevelopmental outcomes.[24] Recently, the contribution of nonprotein calories to linear growth and lean body mass has also been noted. Improved energy intake during hospitalization is associated with increased FFM accretion at 4 months corrected age, and improved linear growth out to 24 months corrected age for prematurity.[7,9] In addition, findings of improved FFM accretion with increased caloric goals (150–160 kcal/kg/d) have not been coupled with increases in fat mass during the hospitalization or in short-term follow-up.[9,38] Specific fats are also important for protein accretion. Similar to branch-chain amino acids, long-chain polyunsaturated fatty acids are potent signaling molecules that affect the expression of genes and, thus, proteins that control cell growth and differentiation.[46] Therefore, current evidence does not support limiting energy intake as a prudent method of normalizing body composition by reducing fat accretion. Such a strategy may in fact reduce linear growth and lean body mass.

Zinc, second only to iron in trace-metal abundance in the brain, plays a key role in a variety of functions that regulate linear and brain growth. These functions include gene expression, enzyme and growth factor (IGF-1) activity, neurogenesis, cell signaling, and modulation of neurotransmitter activity in the developing brain.[47] Most research related to zinc and brain development has been done in rodent models. Mild zinc deficiency during gestation leads to learning and memory deficits in pups.[48] Several studies have shown that zinc supplementation, in the setting of malnutrition, leads to improvement in biochemical alterations, in addition to improved growth and behavioral tests.[49,50] Given that zinc is involved in cell replication and is essential for nucleic acid and protein synthesis, it is an extremely important nutrient during periods of rapid brain growth, such as during the third trimester in humans. Clinical studies of zinc supplementation in VLBW infants and other growth-restricted populations show a significant impact on linear growth[51–53] and motor scores during infancy.[52]

ROLE OF INFLAMMATION/ILLNESS IN LINEAR GROWTH AND BRAIN DEVELOPMENT

The complete set of mechanisms responsible for linear-growth suppression, reduced FFM, increased fat mass, and abnormal fat distribution in VLBW preterm infants are not understood, and represent a significant gap in knowledge that prevents optimal clinical management. In previous studies, growth failure has been proposed to be primarily, if not exclusively, due to a lack of nutritional intake.[54] However, several studies have suggested that weight gain during hospitalization is also negatively influenced by acute and chronic illnesses affecting preterm infants, including sepsis, necrotizing enterocolitis, and bronchopulmonary dysplasia. In the past these findings were interpreted to mean that these medical conditions limit the practitioner's ability to provide adequate nutritional intake.[55–57]

More recently, the relationship of nonnutritional factors, including inflammation, to linear growth/FFM accretion in preterm infants has been considered. Degree of illness and inflammation have been shown to be negatively associated with the degree of catch-up growth in weight, length, and FFM domains after discharge in preterm infants.[7,9] In particular, associations of these nonnutritional factors in the NICU with subsequent linear growth persist until at least 24 months corrected age.[7] These associations with illness implicate inflammatory cytokine activation in the etiology of reduced linear and FFM growth rate. In addition, the long-term nature of altered growth and body composition suggests that longer-term disturbances in regulation of the GH/IGF-1 axis have occurred and cannot be attributed solely to inadequate protein and energy intake, which have largely resolved by the time of hospital discharge. Critically ill children and adults become relatively GH resistant, with elevated GH levels and inappropriately low IGF-1 levels.[58,59] In turn, the GH axis is suppressed by inflammation. In studies of children with chronic inflammation, levels of interleukin (IL)-6 and tumor necrosis factor (TNF)-α have been associated with diminished IGF-1 levels and poor linear growth.[60] Immune activation, as measured by C-reactive protein, has been shown to correlate with decreased linear growth in a population of stunted children,[61] but associations have not yet been examined in the preterm population.

Inflammatory markers have been implicated in neuroinflammation, and have been shown to have negative effects on cognition and, specifically, memory.[62] Increased IL-8 and TNF-α levels have been associated with neurodevelopmental impairment, cerebral palsy, and Mental Developmental Index and Psychomotor Developmental Index of less than 70 in preterm infants.[63] Adipose tissue produces and releases several proinflammatory and anti-inflammatory factors, including leptin, TNF-α, IL-6, and adiponectin.[64] Altered levels of these molecules have been observed in a variety of inflammatory conditions, and have been shown to cross the blood-brain barrier and potentially affect cognition.[65–67] The relationship between increased adiposity and levels of these adipokines has not yet been explored in preterm infants; however, knowledge of this relationship may allow a better understanding of the mechanisms linking altered adiposity, FFM accretion/linear growth, and cognition.

LINEAR GROWTH/FFM GAINS AND NEURODEVELOPMENTAL OUTCOMES

Diminished linear growth, irrespective of weight gain, is common in VLBW preterm infants until 24 months corrected age, and has a significant relationship with reduced cognition.[7] Even when controlling for weight and head circumference z-scores, cognitive scores at 24 months corrected age are positively related to linear growth in the first year after discharge, with an increase of approximately 4 points for each 1 SD increase in length z-score. Similarly, language scores on the Bayley Scales of Infant Development (BSID)-III at 24 months corrected age are positively related to linear growth from birth to hospital discharge, with an improvement of approximately 8 points for each 1 SD increase in z-score. Recently, a large study of preterm low birth weight infants demonstrated that more rapid linear growth from term to 4 months corrected age is associated with lower odds of IQ being less than 85 at ages 8 and 18 years.[5] In

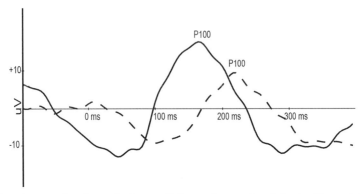

Fig. 2. Grand mean visually evoked potential waveforms of an infant with a relatively low fat-free mass (FFM) at both visits (2.3 g at visit 1 and 4.39 g at visit 2) (*dashed line*) versus an infant with a relatively high FFM at both visits (3.03 g at visit 1 and 5.56 g at visit 2) (*solid line*). (*From* Pfister KM, Gray HL, Miller NC, et al. An exploratory study of the relationship of fat-free mass to speed of brain processing in preterm infants. Pediatr Res 2013;74(5):576–83; with permission.)

addition, improved linear growth after hospital discharge in a group of infants born at less than 33 weeks' gestation is associated with improved motor scores at 18 months corrected age on the BSID-II.[6] Improved postnatal catch-up linear growth in VLBW infants in Switzerland is associated with improved cognitive and motor scores and lower rates of cerebral palsy at 2 years corrected age.[68] Similar correlations have also been noted in institutionalized children in Romania and children in Thailand, who demonstrate a pattern of growth failure that is also characterized by greater length rather than weight suppression.[69,70]

Improved FFM accretion has also recently been linked to improved cognitive development.[25] In a small group of preterm infants, increased FFM at term and 4 months corrected age was associated with faster neuronal processing measured using visual evoked potentials at 4 months corrected age (**Fig. 2**).

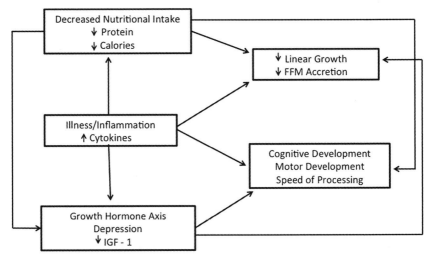

Fig. 3. The complex interactions between nutrition, inflammation, linear growth, and development. FFM, fat-free mass; IGF-1, insulin-like growth factor 1.

These associations of linear growth/FFM gains and later cognition may be explained by the known positive effects of protein status on neuronal growth and differentiation, as evidenced by studies assessing the consequences of protein restriction. However, the primary neuropathology likely results from a lack of protein accretion, which may be due to lack of protein intake or increased protein breakdown. Premature infants are at risk for both low protein intake and inflammatory states that promote protein breakdown. Thus, medical conditions such as inflammatory states that increase somatic protein breakdown are likely to result in protein deficits similar to those noted with dietary restriction (**Fig. 3**). Understanding the role of this axis warrants further study, as IGF-1 and GH have been found to be neuroprotective and neurostimulatory in animal models as well as in healthy children, and support a link between gains in lean body mass and cognitive development.[45,71,72]

SUMMARY

Evidence suggests that diminished linear growth and FFM gains are potentially important markers of future cognitive deficit in VLBW preterm infants. Possibly this is due to associations with reduced GH-axis activation (lower IGF-1), which may reduce myelination and synaptic density, and may be influenced by both nutritional and nonnutritional factors. Optimization of nutrition, including protein intake, in addition to decreasing the duration or frequency of inflammatory episodes, will likely improve long-term outcomes. Additional strategies of possible GH or IGF-1 supplementation should be considered, and need further investigation.

REFERENCES

1. Hamilton BE, Hoyert DL, Martin JA, et al. Annual summary of vital statistics: 2010-2011. Pediatrics 2013;131(3):548–58.
2. Stoll BJ, Hansen NI, Bell EF, et al. Neonatal outcomes of extremely preterm infants from the NICHD Neonatal Research Network. Pediatrics 2010;126(3): 443–56.
3. Hack M, Schluchter M, Cartar L, et al. Growth of very low birth weight infants to age 20 years. Pediatrics 2003;112(1 Pt 1):e30–8. Available at: http://www.ncbi. nlm.nih.gov/pubmed/12837903. Accessed December 11, 2013.
4. Reichman B, Chessex P, Putet G, et al. Diet, fat accretion, and growth in premature infants. N Engl J Med 1981;305(25):1495–500.
5. Belfort MB, Gillman MW, Buka SL, et al. Preterm infant linear growth and adiposity gain: trade-offs for later weight status and intelligence quotient. J Pediatr 2013;163(6):1564–9.e2.
6. Belfort MB, Rifas-Shiman SL, Sullivan T, et al. Infant growth before and after term: effects on neurodevelopment in preterm infants. Pediatrics 2011;128: e899–906. http://dx.doi.org/10.1542/peds.2011-0282.
7. Ramel SE, Demerath EW, Gray HL, et al. The relationship of poor linear growth velocity with neonatal illness and two year neurodevelopment in preterm infants. Neonatology 2012;102:19–24.
8. Johnson MJ, Wootton SA, Leaf AA, et al. Preterm birth and body composition at term equivalent age: a systematic review and meta-analysis. Pediatrics 2012; 130(3):E640–9. http://dx.doi.org/10.1542/peds.2011-3379.
9. Ramel SE, Gray H, Larson Ode K, et al. Body composition changes in preterm infants following hospital discharge: a comparison to term infants. J Pediatr Gastroenterol Nutr 2011;53(3):333–8.

10. Liotto N, Garbarino F, Garavaglia E, et al. Growth and body composition changes in late preterm infants in the first months of life. Pediatr Med Chir 2013;35(4):172–6.

11. American Academy of Pediatrics, Committee on Nutrition. Nutritional needs of low-birth-weight infants. Pediatrics 1985;75:976–86.

12. Martin CR, Brown YF, Ehrenkranz RA, et al. Nutritional practices and growth velocity in the first month of life in extremely premature infants. Pediatrics 2009; 124(2):649–57.

13. Franz AR, Pohlandt F, Bode H, et al. Intrauterine, early neonatal, and postdischarge growth and neurodevelopmental outcome at 5.4 years in extremely preterm infants after intensive neonatal nutritional support. Pediatrics 2009;123: e101–9. http://dx.doi.org/10.1542/peds.2008-1352.

14. Ehrenkranz RA, Dusick AM, Vohr BR, et al. Growth in the neonatal intensive care unit influences neurodevelopmental and growth outcomes of extremely low birth weight infants. Pediatrics 2006;117:1253–61.

15. Cooke R, Lucas A, Yudkin P, et al. Head circumference as an index of brain weight in the fetus and newborn. Early Hum Dev 1977;1(2):145–9.

16. Cheong JL, Hunt RW, Anderson PJ, et al. Head growth in preterm infants: correlation with magnetic resonance imaging and neurodevelopmental outcome. Pediatrics 2008;121:e1534–40. http://dx.doi.org/10.1542/peds.2007-2671.

17. Snijders RJ, Nicolaides KH. Fetal biometry at 14-40 weeks' gestation. Ultrasound Obstet Gynecol 1994;4(1):34–48.

18. Vinall J, Grunau RE, Brant R, et al. Slower postnatal growth is associated with delayed cerebral cortical maturation in preterm newborns. Sci Transl Med 2013;5(168):168ra8. http://dx.doi.org/10.1126/scitranslmed.3004666.

19. Neubauer V, Griesmaier E, Pehböck-Walser N, et al. Poor postnatal head growth in very preterm infants is associated with impaired neurodevelopment outcome. Acta Paediatr 2013;102(9):883–8.

20. Forbes GB. Stature and lean body mass. Am J Clin Nutr 1974;27(6):595–602.

21. Forbes GB. Relation of lean body mass to height in children and adolescents. Pediatr Res 1972;6:32–7.

22. Skullerud K. Variations in the size of the human brain. Influences of age, sex, body mass index, alcoholism, Alzheimer changes and cerebral atherosclerosis. Acta Neurol Scand Suppl 1985;102:1–94.

23. Lubchenco LO, Hansman C, Boyd E. Intrauterine growth in length and head circumference as estimated from live births at gestational ages from 26 to 42 weeks. Pediatrics 1966;37:403–8.

24. Stephens BE, Walden RV, Gargus RA, et al. First-week protein and energy intakes are associated with 18-month developmental outcomes in extremely low birth weight infants. Pediatrics 2009;123:1337–43.

25. Pfister KM, Gray HL, Miller NC, et al. An exploratory study of the relationship of fat-free mass to speed of brain processing in preterm infants. Pediatr Res 2013; 74(5):576–83.

26. Kuzawa CW. Adipose tissue in human infancy and childhood: an evolutionary perspective. Am J Phys Anthropol 1998;27:177–209.

27. Roggero P, Giannì ML, Amato O, et al. Is term newborn body composition being achieved postnatally in preterm infants? Early Hum Dev 2009;85:349–52.

28. Giannì ML, Roggero P, Taroni F, et al. Adiposity in small for gestational age preterm infants assessed at term equivalent age. Arch Dis Child Fetal Neonatal Ed 2009;94:F368–72.

29. Uthaya S, Thomas EL, Hamilton G, et al. Altered adiposity after extremely preterm birth. Pediatr Res 2005;57(2):211–5.

30. van Goudoever JB, Sulkers EJ, Lafeber HN, et al. Short-term growth and substrate use in very-low-birth-weight infants fed formulas with different energy contents. Am J Clin Nutr 2000;71:816–21.
31. Kashyap S, Schulze KF, Forsyth M, et al. Growth, nutrient retention, and metabolic response in low birth weight infants fed varying intakes of protein and energy. J Pediatr 1988;113:713–21.
32. Kretchmer N, Beard JL, Carlson S. The role of nutrition in the development of normal cognition. Am J Clin Nutr 1996;63(6):997S–1001S.
33. Goldman HI, Goldman J, Kaufman I, et al. Late effects of early dietary protein intake on low-birth-weight-infants. J Pediatr 1974;85(6):764–9.
34. Thureen PJ, Melara D, Fennessey PV, et al. Effect of low versus high intravenous amino acid intake on very low birth weight infants in the early neonatal period. Pediatr Res 2003;53(1):24–32.
35. Poindexter BB, Langer JC, Dusick AM, et al, National Institute of Child Health and Human Development Neonatal Research Network. Early provision of parenteral amino acids in extremely low birth weight infants: relation to growth and neurodevelopmental outcome. J Pediatr 2006;148(3):300–5.
36. Isaacs EB, Gadian DG, Sabatini S, et al. The effect of early human diet on caudate volumes and IQ. Pediatr Res 2008;63(3):308–14.
37. Biasini A, Marvulli L, Neri E, et al. Growth and neurological outcome in ELBW preterms fed with human milk and extra-protein supplementation as routine practice: do we need further evidence? J Matern Fetal Neonatal Med 2012;25(Suppl 4):72–4.
38. Costa-Orvay JA, Figueras-Aloy J, Romera G, et al. The effects of varying protein and energy intakes on the growth and body composition of very low birth weight infants. Nutr J 2011;10:140.
39. Fuglestad A, Rao R, Georgieff M. The role of nutrition in cognitive development. In: Nelson CA, Luciana L, editors. Handbook of developmental cognitive neuroscience. 2nd edition. Cambridge (MA): MIT Press; 2008. p. 623–42.
40. Peterson BS, Vohr B, Staib LH. Regional brain volume abnormalities and long-term cognitive outcome in preterm infants. JAMA 2000;284(15):1939–47.
41. Davis EP, Buss C, Muftuler LT, et al. Children's brain development benefits from longer gestation. Front Psychol 2011;2:1. http://dx.doi.org/10.3389/fpsyg.2011.00001.
42. Fretham SJ, Carlson ES, Georgieff MK. The role of iron in learning and memory. Adv Nutr 2011;2:112–21.
43. Ketelslegers JM, Maiter D, Maes M, et al. Nutritional regulation of insulin-like growth factor-I. Metabolism 1995;44(10 Suppl 4):50–7.
44. Shambaugh GE 3rd, Natarajan N, Davenport ML, et al. Nutritional insult and recovery in the neonatal rat cerebellum: insulin-like growth factors (IGFs) and their binding proteins (IGFBPs). Neurochem Res 1995;20:475–90.
45. Hansen-Pupp I, Hövel H, Löfqvist C, et al. Circulatory insulin-like growth factor-I and brain volumes in relation to neurodevelopmental outcome in very preterm infants. Pediatr Res 2013;74(5):564–9.
46. Uauy R, Dangour AD. Nutrition in brain development and aging: role of essential fatty acids. Nutr Rev 2006;64(5):S24–33.
47. Gower-Winter SD, Levenson CW. Zinc in the central nervous system: from molecules to behavior. Biofactors 2011;38(3):186–93.
48. Halas ES, Hunt CD, Eberhardt MJ. Learning and memory disabilities in young adult rats from mildly zinc deficient dams. Physiol Behav 1986;37:451–8.

49. Ladd FV, Ladd AA, Ribeiro AA, et al. Zinc and glutamine improve brain development in suckling mice subjected to early postnatal malnutrition. Nutrition 2010;26(6):662–70.

50. Adebayo OL, Adenuga GA, Sandhir R. Postnatal protein malnutrition induces neurochemical alterations leading to behavioral deficits in rats: prevention by selenium or zinc supplementation. Nutr Neurosci 2013 [Epub ahead of print]. Available at: http://www.ncbi.nlm.nih.gov/pubmed/24144002. Accessed December 11, 2013.

51. Ram Kumar TV, Ramji S. Effect of zinc supplementation on growth in very low birth weight infants. J Trop Pediatr 2012;58(1):50–4.

52. Friel JK, Andrews WL, Matthew JD, et al. Zinc supplementation in very-low-birth-weight infants. J Pediatr Gastroenterol Nutr 1993;17(1):97–104.

53. Imdad A, Bhutta ZA. Effect of preventive zinc supplementation on linear growth in children under 5 years of age in developing countries: a meta-analysis of studies for input to the lives saved tool. BMC Public Health 2011;11(Suppl 3): S22. http://dx.doi.org/10.1186/1471-2458-11-S3-S22.

54. Embleton NE, Pang N, Cooke RJ. Postnatal malnutrition and growth retardation: an inevitable consequence of current recommendations in preterm infants? Pediatrics 2001;107:270–3.

55. Ehrenkranz RA. Growth outcomes of very low-birth weight infants in the newborn intensive care unit. Clin Perinatol 2000;27(2):324–45.

56. Marks KA, Reichman B, Lusky A, et al, Israel Neonatal Network. Fetal growth and postnatal growth failure in very-low-birthweight infants. Acta Paediatr 2006;95(2):236–42.

57. Berry MA, Abrahamowicz M, Usher RH. Factors associated with growth of extremely premature infants during initial hospitalization. Pediatrics 1997; 100(4):640–6.

58. Gardelis JG, Hatzis TD, Stamogiannou LN, et al. Activity of the growth hormone/insulin-like growth factor-1 axis in critically ill children. J Pediatr Endocrinol Metab 2005;18(4):363–72.

59. Gelato MC. The growth hormone/insulin-like growth factor axis in critical illness. J Pediatr Endocrinol Metab 2000;13:1023–9.

60. Ballinger A. Fundamental mechanisms of growth failure in inflammatory bowel disease. Horm Res 2002;58(Suppl 1):7–10.

61. McDade TW, Reyes-García V, Tanner S, et al. Maintenance versus growth: investigating the costs of immune activation among children in lowland Bolivia. Am J Phys Anthropol 2008;136(4):478–84.

62. Belarbi K, Jopson T, Tweedie D, et al. TNF-α protein synthesis inhibitor restores neuronal function and reverses cognitive deficits induced by chronic neuroinflammation. J Neuroinflammation 2012;9:23. http://dx.doi.org/10.1186/1742-2094-9-23.

63. Carlo WA, McDonald SA, Tyson JE, et al. Cytokines and neurodevelopmental outcomes in extremely low birth weight infants. J Pediatr 2011;159(6): 919–925e.3. http://dx.doi.org/10.1016/j.jpeds.2011.05.042.

64. Fantuzzi G. Adipose tissue, adipokines, and inflammation. J Allergy Clin Immunol 2005;115(5):911–9.

65. Banks WA. Role of the blood-brain barrier in the evolution of feeding and cognition. Ann N Y Acad Sci 2012;1264(1):13–9.

66. Harvey J, Shanley LJ, O'Malley D, et al. Leptin: a potential cognitive enhancer? Biochem Soc Trans 2005;33(5):1029–32.

67. Paz-Filho GJ, Babikian T, Asarnow R, et al. Leptin replacement improves cognitive development. PLoS One 2008;3(8):e3098. http://dx.doi.org/10.1371/journal.pone.0003098.

68. Latal-Hajnal B, von Siebenthal K, Kovari H, et al. Postnatal growth in VLBW infants: significant association with neurodevelopmental outcome. J Pediatr 2003;143(2):163–7.
69. Pongcharoen T, Ramakrishnan U, DiGirolamo AM, et al. Influence of prenatal and postnatal growth on intellectual functioning in school-aged children. Arch Pediatr Adolesc Med 2012;166(5):411–6.
70. Johnson DE, Guthrie D, Smyke AT, et al. Growth and associations between auxology, caregiving environment, and cognition in socially deprived Romanian children randomized to foster vs. ongoing institutional care. Arch Pediatr Adolesc Med 2010;164(6):507–16.
71. Scheepens A, Möderscheim T, Gluckman PD. The role of growth hormone in neural development. Horm Res 2005;64(Suppl 3):66–72.
72. Gunnell D, Miller LL, Rogers I, et al. Association of insulin-like growth factor and insulin-like growth factor-binding protein-3 with intelligence quotient among 8 to 9-year old children in the Avon longitudinal study of parents and children. Pediatrics 2005;116(5):e681–6. http://dx.doi.org/10.1542/peds.2004-2390.

Protein Intake and Neurodevelopmental Outcomes

Bonnie E. Stephens, MD[a,b,*], Betty R. Vohr, MD[c]

KEYWORDS

- Protein • Neonatal • Prematurity • Outcomes • Neurodevelopment

KEY POINTS

- Biologic factors associated with prematurity impede the ability to achieve current recommended protein intake for preterm infants in the first week of life.
- Recognition of potential deleterious effects of nutritional deprivation among extremely preterm infants has resulted in recommendations for increased parenteral amino acid intake.
- There is evidence of benefit of early protein intake on head circumference growth among preterm infants.
- Further studies are needed to clarify the relationships among early protein intake, early head growth and neurodevelopmental outcomes, and the differential effects of gender.

There is a continuously accumulating body of evidence that suggests that malnutrition during critical periods of brain growth and development alters the growth trajectory of the developing brain and can have permanent negative developmental consequences.[1–3] Although a great deal of indirect evidence points to the importance of protein intake for the developing brain, there still exists very little direct evidence of the effects of protein intake on neurodevelopment.

In humans, the most critical developmental period of brain growth and function occurs during the third trimester of pregnancy and the first 2 years of postnatal life.[1,4] During this period, brain growth and development are occurring more rapidly than at any other time in life. At 20 weeks' gestation, the brain weighs only 10% of what it weighs at term and is completely smooth, with only the Sylvian fissure having

The authors have no conflicts of interest to disclose.

[a] Department of Pediatrics, Warren Alpert Medical School, Brown University, 222 Richmond Street, Providence, RI, USA; [b] NICU, Community Medical Center, 2827 Fort Missoula Road, Missoula, MT 59804, USA; [c] Neonatal Follow-up Program, Women and Infants Hospital, Department of Pediatrics, Warren Alpert Medical School, Brown University, 222 Richmond Street, Providence, RI, USA

* Corresponding author. NICU, Community Medical Center, 2827 Fort Missoula Road, Missoula, MT 59804.

E-mail address: bstephens@communitymed.org

formed. The brain increases in weight in a linear fashion from 20 to 40 weeks, and in the process, develops all remaining gyri and sulci.[5] The volume of the cortical gray matter increases 4-fold from 29 to 40 weeks' gestation, and a 5-fold increase in white matter volume occurs from 35 to 40 weeks.[6] In addition to neuron formation, migration, maturation, synapse formation, and pruning via apoptosis are all occurring rapidly during this period and continue to occur throughout and beyond the neonatal period. The rapid changes associated with these developmental processes make the developing brain extremely vulnerable to environmental perturbations.[1,4]

One such environmental perturbation with the potential to have lasting effects on the developing brain is an alteration in nutritional intake. In studies of malnutrition in rat pups, even mild malnutrition during this "critical period" in brain development, resulting from a larger than normal litter size, led to deficits in neuron formation in the cerebellar granular layer and deeper layers of the cerebral cortex.[1] In preterm human infants with birth weights less than 1750 g, caloric deprivation (defined as intakes of <85 kcal/kg/d) has been directly related to poor head growth, and prolonged periods of caloric deprivation (greater than 4 weeks in duration) has been associated with lower scores on the Bayley Psychomotor Developmental Index (PDI) at 12 months of age.[7]

Thus, the provision of adequate nutrition to infants during the neonatal period seems to be critical. Despite this, nutritional practices vary greatly among neonatal intensive care units (NICUs), and energy-containing macronutrients (protein, carbohydrate, and lipid) have historically been introduced slowly and increased cautiously because of concerns for intolerance. This intolerance results in a period of nutritional deficiency that is common and accepted as inevitable for newborns hospitalized in the NICU.[8,9] Although all hospitalized newborns are vulnerable, those born preterm are the most vulnerable and the most studied in the published literature.

The precise nutritional needs of the preterm infant are still unknown, as are the duration and degree of undernutrition that places the infant at neurodevelopmental risk. The American Academy of Pediatrics Committee on Nutrition recognizes the importance of adequate nutrition for these vulnerable infants and recommends providing sufficient energy and nutrients to meet the requirements of the growing fetus with the goal of "approximating the rate of growth and composition of weight gain for a normal fetus at the same postmenstrual age."[10,11] Nevertheless, there are several challenges encountered when attempting to achieve nutrient intake in preterm infants commensurate with the intrauterine environment. Gastrointestinal constraints result in delays in achieving full enteral feeds. Small stomach capacity, slow gastric emptying, decreased intestinal motility, decreased enzyme production, immature sucking, and diminished suck-swallow coordination contribute to potential nutritional deficits associated with enteral feeds. Ehrenkranz and colleagues[12] showed that age of first enteral feed was inversely related to birth weight. Parenteral alimentation, therefore, is the initial primary method for providing early nutrition, including protein to very preterm infants, and even with the provision of parenteral nutrition, there remains a difference between the nutrient supply that the normally growing fetus typically receives and that received by the postnatal, preterm counterpart.

The composition of the nutrients delivered by the placenta reflects the unique needs of the growing fetus. Glucose is delivered at a rate that reflects energy use; amino acid uptake is high and far exceeds that needed for accretion (oxidation of the excess is used as a significant energy source), and lipid uptake is minimal. The typical neonate in the intensive care unit receives high rates of glucose and lipid infusion in an attempt to provide adequate calories for growth, yet lower of rates amino acid/protein infusion.[13,14] This practice of limiting protein intake is especially commonplace in the treatment of the sick or extremely low-birth-weight neonates during the early neonatal period, in an attempt to avoid potential side effects, such as azotemia or acidosis, seen with the infusion of some amino acid solutions. Thus, nutritional deficits inevitably occur.[8] These deficits are greatest in the first week of life but continue to accumulate through the first month.

In the typical fetus at less than 32 weeks, rates of protein accretion are approximately 2 g per day.[15] In contrast, when infants receive an intravenous infusion of dextrose alone, rates of protein loss in the stable, 32-week preterm infant are ~1 g/kg/d and in the extremely preterm infant (26 weeks) approach 1.5 g/kg/d.[16] Thus, cumulatively, the extremely preterm infant receiving glucose alone loses 1% to 2% of their protein stores daily.[16] When placed on an amino acid infusion rate of 1.1 g/kg/d, protein balance is zero, with no losses, but also no protein accretion to support growth and development.[17] At infusion rates of at least 1.5 g/kg/d, protein balance becomes positive, and some protein accretion begins to occur. However, even at infusion rates of 3 g/kg/d, protein accretion remains less than that of the reference fetus. Adequate accretion rates require infusion rates of 3.85 g/kg/d if the goal remains to "approximate the rate of growth and composition of weight gain for a normal fetus at the same postmenstrual age."[16] Provision of less results in cumulative losses that are difficult to make up. For example, the infant who receives only 2 g/kg/d of amino acid infusion develops a net loss of 14 g/kg over the course of a week.[8] Infusion of only 3 g/kg/d still results in a net loss of almost 6 g/kg at the end of the first week of life.

Why has the fear of side effects kept us from providing adequate protein to our vulnerable preterm infants? Historically, the amino acid solutions available to us were casein hydrolysates, which often led to acidosis and hyperammonemia. However, since the 1980s, newer crystalline formulations have been available that reduce the incidence and severity of negative consequences.

There is clinical evidence that parenteral protein can be provided safely, without adverse clinical sequelae, in the early neonatal period.[18–23] Rates of acidosis and elevated blood urea nitrogen (BUN) levels are similar regardless of early protein administration.[18–23] In fact, there is no correlation between amino acid intake in the early neonatal period and serum BUN levels.[24] Amino acid levels also remain safely at or below levels of the reference fetus during amino acid infusions.[22] Even parenteral amino acid intake of 3 to 3.5 in the first days of life has been shown to be both safe and effective in improving protein accretion.[19,22]

Higher protein (and calorie) intakes, even in the first days of life, result in better growth at NICU discharge in very-low-birth-weight (<1500 g) infants. Three studies have demonstrated lower rates of growth restriction (parameters <10%) at discharge in those infants fed more protein and calories in the first weeks of life.[20,23,25] A 2013 Cochrane Review of trials examining early (<24 hours) versus late (≥24 hours) parenteral amino acid administration in premature infants on outcome at 28 days identified improved nitrogen balance but no effect on length and head circumference.[26] The trials in this review were limited by small sample size. Neurodevelopmental outcomes were not reported in any of these studies.

An association between poor growth and neurodevelopmental outcome has been demonstrated in other studies. Connors and colleagues[27] demonstrated an association between lower developmental scores and weight less than the 10th percentile at 2 years of age, in a cohort of 70 high-risk, extremely low-birth-weight infants. Ehrenranz and colleagues[28] demonstrated a significant relationship between in-hospital growth velocity and neurodevelopmental outcome in 490 extremely low-birth-weight infants. Lower rate of weight gain and lower rate of head growth were both significantly associated with cerebral palsy, Bayley Mental Developmental Index (MDI) less than

70, and neurodevelopmental impairment at 18-months corrected age, when controlling for confounding variables. However, neither of these studies examined nutrient intake.

Poor in utero and extrauterine head growth in very-low-birth-weight infants has also been shown to predict lower scores on the MDI at 15 to 20 months of age,[29,30] and lower verbal and performance intelligence quotients (IQ), receptive and expressive language, and academic abilities at school age.[31] In infants born small for gestational age, head circumference "catch-up" growth has been correlated with higher energy intake during the first 10 days of life and higher IQ later in life,[32] thus implying an indirect association between intake and neurodevelopmental outcome.

Interpretation of results of protein administration trials may be confounded by the degree to which centers achieve successful implementation of the nutrition protocol. The Glutamine trial[33] randomized infants weighing 401 to 1000 g, receiving parenteral nutrition within 72 hours of birth, to receive either TrophAmine (control) or an isonitrogenous study amino acid solution with 20% glutamine for up to 120 days of age, death, or discharge from the hospital. No group differences were found in rates of death, late-onset sepsis, or growth at 36 weeks. However, examination of the data indicated that only 18% of infants received the parenteral protein ordered.

Poindexter and colleagues[34] reanalyzed the growth data from the Glutamine Trial in a secondary analysis and demonstrated better head growth at 18-months corrected age in a cohort of extremely low-birth-weight infants (<1000 g) who actually received at least 3 g/kg/d of amino acids in the first 5 days of life, compared with those who received less. Significantly more infants in the group who received less than 3 g/kg/d in the first 5 days had a head circumference less than the 10% and/or less than the 5%. In addition, boys who did not receive 3 g/kg/d of amino acids in the first 5 days of life had smaller head circumferences. There was no effect for girls. No differences in rates of neurodevelopmental impairment (MDI <70, PDI <70, cerebral palsy, blind, deaf) at 18-months corrected age were identified between infants receiving higher or lower protein intakes. Thus, better head growth did not translate to better neurodevelopmental outcomes.

To date, only one published study examines the direct association between protein intake in the first week of life and neurodevelopmental outcomes.[35] This study analyzed the total daily enteral and parenteral calorie and protein intake in all extremely low-birth-weight survivors in a single NICU during a 2-year period and found a significant association between intake and 18-month neurodevelopmental outcome. Every gram per kilogram per day of protein received in the first week of life was associated with an 8.2-point increase in MDI score at 18 months. However, this was a retrospective analysis and rates of amino acid infusion were low, with an average of only 1 g/kg/d on the first day of life and a gradual increase to 2.9 g/kg/d by the end of the first week.

A prospective longitudinal study is needed to examine the effects of early, higher parenteral protein intake fully in conjunction with known confounders on the outcomes of preterm infants. At least one such trial is currently underway.

A clear association between early enteral intake and neurodevelopmental outcome has been demonstrated in larger preterm infants. Lucas and colleagues[36,37] demonstrated higher cognitive and motor scores at 18-month corrected age, as well as higher verbal IQs and lower rates of cerebral palsy at 7.5 to 8 years of age in preterm infants (<1850 g) fed preterm formula containing 2 g protein and 80 kcal per deciliter versus term formula containing 1.45 g protein and 68 kcal per deciliter for the first 4 weeks of life. This association was most pronounced in infants born small for gestational age. The association with verbal IQ persisted at 16-year follow-up.[38]

The association between breast milk intake and neurodevelopmental outcome is less clear, especially in smaller preterm infants. Furman and colleagues[39] demonstrated no effect of maternal milk intake in the first 4 weeks of life on 20-month cognitive or motor outcomes in a cohort of 98 very-low-birth-weight infants (<1500 g). Conversely, in a cohort of 1035 extremely low-birth-weight infants, Vohr and colleagues[40] found that those infants fed more breast milk during hospitalization in the NICU had higher 18-month MDI scores.

Studies of enteral nutrition and its effects on developmental outcome fail to account for nutrition in the first days and weeks of life, because most extremely low-birth-weight infants do not begin to feed enterally for several days and do not reach full enteral feedings for weeks. In addition, although preterm human milk has a higher protein level than term human milk,[41] protein and energy levels are still inadequate for growth, and supplementation with human milk fortifiers is needed.[42,43]

In summary, there remains limited evidence in regard to the neurodevelopmental effects of protein intake in the neonatal period. However, the evidence for higher levels of enteral protein intake, combined with the indirect and retrospective data on parenteral protein intake, supports the concept that adequate protein intake in the hospitalized preterm infant may be associated with better neurodevelopmental outcomes.

REFERENCES

1. Dobbing J, Sands J. Vulnerability of developing brain. IX. The effect of nutritional growth retardation on the timing of the brain growth-spurt. Biol Neonate 1971;19: 363–78.
2. Levitsky DA, Strupp BJ. Malnutrition and the brain: changing concepts, changing concerns. J Nutr 1995;125:2212S–20S.
3. Thureen PJ, Hay WW Jr. Early aggressive nutrition in preterm infants. Semin Neonatol 2001;6:403–15.
4. Dobbing J, Sands J. Quantitative growth and development of human brain. Arch Dis Child 1973;48:757–67.
5. Guihard-Costa AM, Larroche JC. Differential growth between the fetal brain and its infratentorial part. Early Hum Dev 1990;23:27–40.
6. Huppi PS, Warfield S, Kikinis R, et al. Quantitative magnetic resonance imaging of brain development in premature and mature newborns. Ann Neurol 1998;43: 224–35.
7. Georgieff MK, Hoffman JS, Pereira GR, et al. Effect of neonatal caloric deprivation on head growth and 1-year developmental status in preterm infants. J Pediatr 1985;107:581–7.
8. Embleton NE, Pang N, Cooke RJ. Postnatal malnutrition and growth retardation: an inevitable consequence of current recommendations in preterm infants? Pediatrics 2001;107:270–3.
9. Thureen PJ. Early aggressive nutrition in the neonate. Pediatr Rev 1999;20: e45–55.
10. American Academy of Pediatrics, Committee on Nutrition. Nutritional needs of the preterm infant. Pediatric nutrition handbook. Elk Grove Village (IL): American Academy of Pediatrics; 2009. p. 23–54.
11. Tsang RC, Lucas A, Uauy R, et al, editors. Nutritional needs of the preterm infant: scientific basis and practical guidelines. Baltimore (MD): Williams & Wilkins; 1993.
12. Ehrenkranz RA, Younes N, Lemons JA, et al. Longitudinal growth of hospitalized very low birth weight infants. Pediatrics 1999;104:280–9.

13. Carlson SJ, Ziegler EE. Nutrient intakes and growth of very low birth weight infants. J Perinatol 1998;18:252–8.

14. Hay WW. Early postnatal nutritional requirements of the very preterm infant based on a presentation at the NICHD-AAP workshop on research in neonatology. J Perinatol 2006;26(Suppl 2):S13–8.

15. Ziegler EE, O'Donnell AM, Nelson SE, et al. Body composition of the reference fetus. Growth 1976;40:329–41.

16. Denne SC, Poindexter BB. Evidence supporting early nutritional support with parenteral amino acid infusion. Semin Perinatol 2007;31:56–60.

17. van Goudoever JB, Colen T, Wattimena JL, et al. Immediate commencement of amino acid supplementation in preterm infants: effect on serum amino acid concentrations and protein kinetics on the first day of life. J Pediatr 1995;127:458–65.

18. Clark RH, Chace DH, Spitzer AR. Effects of two different doses of amino acid supplementation on growth and blood amino acid levels in premature neonates admitted to the neonatal intensive care unit: a randomized, controlled trial. Pediatrics 2007;120:1286–96.

19. Ibrahim HM, Jeroudi MA, Baier RJ, et al. Aggressive early total parental nutrition in low-birth-weight infants. J Perinatol 2004;24:482–6.

20. Maggio L, Cota F, Gallini F, et al. Effects of high versus standard early protein intake on growth of extremely low birth weight infants. J Pediatr Gastroenterol Nutr 2007;44:124–9.

21. te Braake F, van den Akker CH, Wattimena DJ, et al. Amino acid administration to premature infants directly after birth. J Pediatr 2005;147:457–61.

22. Thureen PJ, Melara D, Fennessey PV, et al. Effect of low versus high intravenous amino acid intake on very low birth weight infants in the early neonatal period. Pediatr Res 2003;53:24–32.

23. Wilson DC, Cairns P, Halliday HL, et al. Randomised controlled trial of an aggressive nutritional regimen in sick very low birthweight infants. Arch Dis Child Fetal Neonatal Ed 1997;77:F4–11.

24. Ridout E, Melara D, Rottinghaus S, et al. Blood urea nitrogen concentration as a marker of amino-acid intolerance in neonates with birthweight less than 1250 g. J Perinatol 2005;25:130–3.

25. Dinerstein A, Nieto RM, Solana CL, et al. Early and aggressive nutritional strategy (parenteral and enteral) decreases postnatal growth failure in very low birth weight infants. J Perinatol 2006;26:436–42.

26. Trivedi A, Sinn JK. Early versus late administration of amino acids in preterm infants receiving parenteral nutrition. Cochrane Database Syst Rev 2013;(7):CD008771.

27. Connors JM, O'Callaghan MJ, Burns YR, et al. The influence of growth on development outcome in extremely low birthweight infants at 2 years of age. J Paediatr Child Health 1999;35:37–41.

28. Ehrenkranz RA, Dusick AM, Vohr BR, et al. Growth in the neonatal intensive care unit influences neurodevelopmental and growth outcomes of extremely low birth weight infants. Pediatrics 2006;117:1253–61.

29. Gross SJ, Oehler JM, Eckerman CO. Head growth and developmental outcome in very low-birth-weight infants. Pediatrics 1983;71:70–5.

30. Hack M, Breslau N, Fanaroff AA. Differential effects of intrauterine and postnatal brain growth failure in infants of very low birth weight. Am J Dis Child 1989;143:63–8.

31. Hack M, Breslau N, Weissman B, et al. Effect of very low birth weight and subnormal head size on cognitive abilities at school age. N Engl J Med 1991;325:231–7.

32. Brandt I, Sticker EJ, Lentze MJ. Catch-up growth of head circumference of very low birth weight, small for gestational age preterm infants and mental development to adulthood. J Pediatr 2003;142:463–8.
33. Poindexter BB, Ehrenkranz RA, Stoll BJ, et al. Parenteral glutamine supplementation does not reduce the risk of mortality or late-onset sepsis in extremely low birth weight infants. Pediatrics 2004;113:1209–15.
34. Poindexter BB, Langer JC, Dusick AM, et al. Early provision of parenteral amino acids in extremely low birth weight infants: relation to growth and neurodevelopmental outcome. J Pediatr 2006;148:300–5.
35. Stephens BE, Walden RV, Gargus RA, et al. First-week protein and energy intakes are associated with 18-month developmental outcomes in extremely low birth weight infants. Pediatrics 2009;123:1337–43.
36. Lucas A, Morley R, Cole TJ. Randomised trial of early diet in preterm babies and later intelligence quotient. BMJ 1998;317:1481–7.
37. Lucas A, Morley R, Cole TJ, et al. Early diet in preterm babies and developmental status at 18 months. Lancet 1990;335:1477–81.
38. Isaacs EB, Morley R, Lucas A. Early diet and general cognitive outcome at adolescence in children born at or below 30 weeks gestation. J Pediatr 2009; 155:229–34.
39. Furman L, Wilson-Costello D, Friedman H, et al. The effect of neonatal maternal milk feeding on the neurodevelopmental outcome of very low birth weight infants. J Dev Behav Pediatr 2004;25:247–53.
40. Vohr BR, Poindexter BB, Dusick AM, et al. Beneficial effects of breast milk in the neonatal intensive care unit on the developmental outcome of extremely low birth weight infants at 18 months of age. Pediatrics 2006;118:e115–23.
41. Bauer J, Gerss J. Longitudinal analysis of macronutrients and minerals in human milk produced by mothers of preterm infants. Clin Nutr 2011;30:215–20.
42. Kashyap S, Schulze KF, Forsyth M, et al. Growth, nutrient retention, and metabolic response of low-birth-weight infants fed supplemented and unsupplemented preterm human milk. Am J Clin Nutr 1990;52:254–62.
43. Premji SS, Fenton TR, Sauve RS. Higher versus lower protein intake in formula-fed low birth weight infants. Cochrane Database Syst Rev 2006;(1):CD003959.

Complications Associated with Parenteral Nutrition in the Neonate

Kara L. Calkins, MD[a],*, Robert S. Venick, MD[b],
Sherin U. Devaskar, MD[a]

KEYWORDS

- Parenteral nutrition • Neonates • Lipids
- Parenteral nutrition–associated liver disease • Infections

KEY POINTS

- Although parenteral nutrition (PN) is life-saving, it is associated with myriad of complications, some of which are transient and others life-threatening, including parenteral nutrition–associated liver disease (PNALD) and central line–associated bloodstream infections (CLABSIs).
- Although fish oil–based lipid emulsions can biochemically reverse PNALD, clinicians should bear in mind that the development and progression of PNALD is multifactorial.
- It remains to be determined whether dose reduction of lipid emulsions can prevent PNALD without sacrificing growth and neurodevelopment.
- The phytosterol, long-chain polyunsaturated fatty acid, and antioxidant content of intravenous lipid products seems to play an important role in the pathogenesis of PNALD.
- Research is needed with regard to optimizing the PN content for the neonatal population so as to safely promote growth and neurodevelopment.

INTRODUCTION

Parental nutrition (PN) is an essential part of the medical management of critically ill neonates. The primary goals of PN are to maintain hydration and electrolyte balance, and to promote growth and neurodevelopment without adverse complications. For a myriad of reasons, up to 70% of neonates in the neonatal intensive care unit (NICU) are prescribed PN at some point, and approximately 16,000 children receive PN in the home setting in the United States (**Box 1**).[1,2] Without PN, children who are unable to consume sufficient enteral nutrition would succumb to malnutrition, dehydration, and electrolyte derangements.

[a] Division of Neonatology and Developmental Biology, Department of Pediatrics, Mattel Children's Hospital, University of California, Los Angeles, Los Angeles, CA, USA; [b] Division of Gastroenterology, Department of Pediatrics, Mattel Children's Hospital, University of California, 10833 Le Conte Avenue, MDCC, Los Angeles, Los Angeles, CA 90095-1752, USA
* Corresponding author.
E-mail address: KCalkins@mednet.ucla.edu

Clin Perinatol 41 (2014) 331–345
http://dx.doi.org/10.1016/j.clp.2014.02.006
0095-5108/14/$ – see front matter © 2014 Elsevier Inc. All rights reserved.

Box 1
Neonatal populations at high risk for complications secondary to parenteral nutrition (PN)

- Premature neonates
  - Feeding intolerance
  - Necrotizing enterocolitis
- Abdominal wall defects
  - Gastroschisis and omphalocele
- Motility disorders
  - Hirschsprung disease and total aganglionosis
- Intestinal obstructions
  - Atresia
  - Pseudo-obstruction
- Malabsorption
  - Surgical short bowel syndrome (ie, necrotizing enterocolitis)
  - Enterocyte disorders (ie, tufting disorders and microvillus inclusion disease)
- Neonates with poor intestinal perfusion
  - Cyanotic congenital heart disease
- Other congenital disorders
  - Congenital diaphragmatic hernia

Although outcomes in poorly resourced countries do not mirror what has been witnessed in well-resourced countries, PN has undoubtedly contributed to the improved survival of infants with gastrointestinal disorders and premature neonates worldwide.[3–6] The survival rate of neonates born in the United States with gastroschisis is approximately 90% to 97%.[7,8] By comparison, mortality rates in poorly resourced countries vary between 40% and 100% depending on surgical and medical treatments including the availability of PN.[3,5] Despite benefits, PN does not come without complications. Whereas some of these complications are transient with recovery, others are associated with an increased risk of morbidity and mortality, specifically parenteral nutrition–associated liver disease (PNALD) and central line–associated bloodstream infections (CLABSIs) (**Fig. 1**).[2] The purpose of this review is to summarize some of the commonly encountered complications associated with PN in the neonatal population.

METABOLIC COMPLICATIONS
Lipid Intolerance

Lipid emulsions provide long-chain polyunsaturated fatty acids (LC-PUFAs), which are important for a multitude of reasons; they maintain the integrity of the cell membrane and serve as precursors to eicosanoids and prostanoids (**Fig. 2**).[9,10] The United States Food and Drug Administration (FDA)-approved and most frequently prescribed intravenous lipid product in the United States, Intralipid® 20% (Frensenius Kabi, Uppsala, Sweden), is derived entirely from soybean oil (SO), which mainly contains omega-6 fatty acids. SO contains the essential LC-PUFAs, linoleic and α-linolenic acid, but lacks the downstream products, arachidonic acid (ARA), eicosapentaenoic acid (EPA), and docosahexaenoic acid (DHA), which are important for cerebral and retinal

Complications of PN
• Metabolic disturbances
• Mechanical issues with the line
• Phlebitis and cellulitis
• Thrombosis
• PNALD
• CLABSIs
• Kidney stones and gallstones
• Metabolic bone disease

Benefits of PN
• Improved nutrition and growth
• Improved neurodevelopment
• LIFE-SAVING

Fig. 1. Common complications and benefits associated with parenteral nutrition (PN). CLABSIs, central line–associated bloodstream infections; PNALD, parenteral nutrition–associated liver disease.

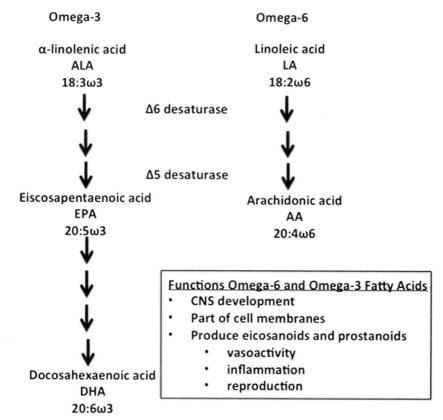

Omega-3

α-linolenic acid
ALA
$18:3\omega3$

Δ6 desaturase

Δ5 desaturase

Eiscosapentaenoic acid
EPA
$20:5\omega3$

Docosahexaenoic acid
DHA
$20:6\omega3$

Omega-6

Linoleic acid
LA
$18:2\omega6$

Arachidonic acid
AA
$20:4\omega6$

Functions Omega-6 and Omega-3 Fatty Acids
• CNS development
• Part of cell membranes
• Produce eicosanoids and prostanoids
• vasoactivity
• inflammation
• reproduction

Fig. 2. Omega-3 and omega-6 fatty acids and their functions. CNS, central nervous system.

development as well as the immune system (see **Fig. 2**, **Table 1**). Owing to increased demand, immature metabolic machinery, and limited stores, it is not surprising that premature neonates and children dependent on parenteral nutrition for a prolonged period are prone to developing omega-6 and omega-3 PUFA deficiencies, which are linked to morbidities such as chronic lung disease and neurodevelopmental impairment.[9,11]

While parenteral lipids serve as an important source of calories, improve metabolic efficiency, and prevent essential fatty acid deficiencies, they can exacerbate or cause hypertriglyceridemia and/or hyperglycemia. Particularly in the face of sepsis, lipids may impair insulin sensitivity and increase gluconeogenesis, and result in lipid and glucose intolerance.[12] The long-term risks of serum hypertriglyceridemia, unlike those for hyperglycemia or hypoglycemia, are unknown.[13–15] The temporary withholding or long-term restriction of lipids also remains controversial.[9,16,17] At the same time, the benefit of providing early and high-dose parenteral lipids shortly after birth is unclear. In 2 meta-analyses, this strategy alone did not appear to decrease common neonatal morbidities.[18,19] However, the prescription of 2 to 3 g/kg/d of parenteral lipids in combination with approximately 2.5 to 3.5 g/kg/d of amino acids at birth may facilitate growth by improving nitrogen balance and anabolism.[20]

Glucose Intolerance

Parenteral glucose infusions, particularly when prescribed at high glucose infusion rates, can result in abnormal serum glucose concentrations. After birth, the incidence of hyperglycemia in the very low birth weight (VLBW) population is inversely proportional to gestational age and birth weight, and can approach an incidence rate of 75%.[13–15] Hyperglycemia and hypoglycemia are associated with increased neonatal morbidity and mortality.[13–15] In the NIRTURE (Neonatal Insulin Replacement Therapy in Europe) study, a multisite, double-blind randomized controlled trial, insulin therapy in the first week of life in VLBW neonates was reported to improve glycemic control and decrease weight loss.[21] However, subjects who received insulin were more likely to become hypoglycemic, die at 28 days of life, and develop ventricular hemorrhage or periventricular lesions in comparison with controls.[21] Interestingly, in a study of neonates with a mean gestational age of 24 weeks, a 60% reduction in the parenteral glucose infusion rate from approximately 8.4 to 3.4 mg/kg/min reduced serum glucose

Table 1 Composition of three different intravenous lipid emulsions			
	Intralipid®	Omegaven®	SMOF®
Vitamin E (mg/L)	38	250	47.6
Phytosterols (mg/L)	343	0	48
Oil Source			
Soybean oil (%)	100	0	30
Fish oil (%)	0	100	15
Coconut oil (%)	0	0	30
Olive oil (%)	0	0	25
Fat Composition			
Linoleic acid (g/100 mL)	5	0.1–0.7	2.85
Arachidonic acid (g/100 mL)	0	0.1–0.4	0.05
α-Linolenic acid (g/100 mL)	0.9	<0.2	0.275
Eicosapentaenoic acid (g/100 mL)	0	1.28–2.82	0.25
Docosahexaenoic acid (g/100 mL)	0	1.44–3.09	0.05

concentrations by 30% without an increased incidence of serum hypoglycemia or change in hepatic gluconeogenesis.[22] In order to combat hyperglycemia, the early introduction of parenteral amino acids has been shown to decrease the risk for hyperglycemia by stimulating endogenous insulin production.[23–27]

Amino Acid–Related Complications

In a double-blind, randomized controlled study by Blanco and colleagues,[25] extremely low birth weight (ELBW, birth weight <1 kg) neonates were assigned to 1 of 2 interventions: early and high-dose amino acids in the form of Aminosyn PF® (Abbott Laboratories, Chicago, IL) or a control dose. The early and high-dose group was prescribed a target goal of approximately 4 g/kg/d by day of life 3, whereas the control group's amino acids were advanced to approximately 3 g/kg/d in the first couple of days of life. In comparison with the control group, the early and high-dose group exhibited decreased growth during follow-up. Whereas neurodevelopmental scores at 18 months postmenstrual age were decreased in the interventional group when compared with controls, at 24 months the cognitive scores were similar between the 2 arms. Of notable concern was the negative correlation discovered between various plasma amino acid concentrations and growth and Mental Developmental Index (MDI).[28,29] It remains unclear as to whether this finding is secondary to the target dose of 4 g/kg/d, with 3 g/kg/d or less in the first few days of life being more appropriate, specific outliers, and/or the specific amino acid formulation. Nevertheless, other studies have not replicated these results and have actually demonstrated the converse. Once a protein and energy deficit occurs, it is difficult to make up. Appropriate provisions of protein and energy promote lean body mass and linear growth–which may be just as important (if not more) as body weight.[24,30,31]

As expected, concentrations of serum blood urea nitrogen (BUN) and, in some subjects, serum ammonia, increased in the early and high-dose amino acid group in comparison with the control group in the aforementioned study by Blanco and colleagues.[20,25,28,29,31] As with hypertriglyceridemia, it remains debatable as to what constitutes a clinically significant state of uremia. What is an appropriate aminogram for VLBW infants, and when parenteral protein should be decreased considering the implications of a protein deficit, also remain questionable.[20,25,27] Higher BUN concentrations are to be expected when clinicians prescribe amino acids at a higher dose immediately after birth, and in most cases reflect amino acid oxidation and protein turnover, not toxicity.

Summary

Although the early introduction of parenteral amino acids and lipids after birth may be associated with transient metabolic complications, numerous studies have demonstrated that PN and continued refinements in PN care have resulted in improved growth and long-term neurodevelopment that have far-researching benefits beyond the NICU.[4,6,24,26,32] Although significant gains have been made, one should remember that neonates, both preterm and term, who depend on PN in the NICU, still have a high rate of growth failure that persists even after hospital discharge.[33,34]

PARENTERAL NUTRITION–ASSOCIATED LIVER DISEASE

Although PN is life-sustaining, it is associated with PNALD, which carries high morbidity and mortality in the pediatric population.[2] PNALD, a heterogeneous liver injury consisting of cholestasis, steatosis, fibrosis, and even cirrhosis, is characteristically defined as the development of persistent, direct hyperbilirubinemia when other causes of liver disease are excluded in patients who have received prolonged courses of PN. As serum direct bilirubin rises, mortality and the need for a small bowel or combined small bowel–liver transplant increases.[1,35] While liver biopsy is considered the gold standard for PNALD diagnosis, this type of invasive surveillance carries risks related to bleeding and anesthesia. As a result, clinicians routinely rely upon laboratory evaluations, specifically serum direct bilirubin concentrations and liver function tests, to monitor PNALD. However, it is well recognized that histological injury begins soon after PN initiation and does not correlate with bilirubin concentrations. In fact, biliirubins can be normal in the presence of severe histological damage.[36]

PNALD risk factors can broadly be characterized as either patient-related or PN-related (**Box 2**). PNALD patient-related risk factors mainly center around the percentage of calories a patient tolerates enterally versus parenterally, which in turn depends on the patient's gastrointestinal function and anatomy, such as length of small-bowel remnant, gastrocolonic continuity, and presence of an ileocecal value. By contemporary analyses, approximately 25% of neonates with gastrointestinal disorders will develop PNALD.[37] The incidence and likelihood of

---

Box 2
Common risk factors for parenteral nutrition–associated liver disease (PNALD)

Patient-Related

- Prematurity
- SGA/IUGR
- Gastrointestinal disorder
- Lack of enteral feeds
- Necrotizing enterocolitis
- Gastrointestinal surgeries, function, and anatomy
  - Bowel length
  - Presence of ileum, ileocecal valve, and colon
  - Intestinal continuity
- Infections

PN-Related

- Prolonged PN duration
- CLABSIs
- Phytosterols
- Type of polyunsaturated fatty acid
- Presence of antioxidants
- Excess or deficiency of macronutrients or micronutrients
  - Carbohydrates
  - Amino acids
  - Fat
  - Copper

Abbreviations: CLABSIs, central line–associated bloodstream infections; IUGR, intrauterine growth restriction; SGA, small for gestational age.

developing PNALD vary by specific gastrointestinal diagnosis and report.[1,37,38] Moreover, PNALD incidence increases significantly when a congenital gastrointestinal diagnosis is complicated by any stage of necrotizing enterocolitis.[1,37–41] For children who develop short bowel syndrome (SBS), 67% will develop PNALD and 17% will progress to end-stage liver failure.[42] In addition, prematurity, birth weight, infections, and perhaps an individual's genetic makeup appear to be important drivers for PNALD.[1,41] The odds ratio for developing cholestasis among neonates with a birth weight of less than 750 g is 13.1, whereas for a neonate with a birth weight between 1 and 1.5 kg this decreases to 2.8.[1] In one study, despite receiving fewer PN days, small for gestational age neonates, in a comparison with appropriate for gestational age controls, had an odds ratio of 3.3 for developing cholestasis.[41]

Intravenous Fatty Acid Emulsions and IFALD

Recent studies have demonstrated that the dose and composition of intravenous fatty acid emulsions may play an important role in the development and progression of PNALD.[16,17,39,40,43,44] SO has been traditionally prescribed at an approximate dose of 0.5 to 4 g/kg/d. The American Academy of Pediatrics recommends a maximum dose of 3 g/kg/d of intravenous lipids. An intravenous lipid emulsion composed entirely of fish oil (FO), commercially available as Omegaven® 10% (Fresenius Kabi, Hamburg, Germany), is composed mainly of the omega-3 fatty acids EPA and DHA (see **Table 1**). FO is not currently FDA-approved but is available outside the United States, and is prescribed at 1 g/kg/d. Studies have provided evidence that when 1 g/kg/d of exclusive FO is substituted for SO, direct hyperbilirubinemia is more likely to resolve, and the incidences of death and transplant may be reduced.[44–46] European studies have also demonstrated that mixed fatty acid emulsions, such as SMOF® (Fresenius Kabi, Hamburg, Germany), which contain soybean, fish, olive, and coconut oils, are associated with improved liver function, decreased markers of inflammation and oxidative injury, and increased antioxidant activity (see **Table 1**).[47–50] Whereas FO and products containing FO appear to biochemically reverse PNALD, their effect on histology, which is equally (if not more) important, remains unknown.[36]

There is also evidence that the incidence and progression of PNALD can be modified by decreasing the SO dose alone.[16,40,51] When compared with a historical cohort who received the standard SO dose, surgical neonates with cholestasis who received 1 g/kg of SO twice a week had an increased incidence of cholestasis resolution (42% vs 10%). However, 8 of 13 neonates developed a triene:tetraene ratio of greater than 0.05 but less than 0.2, and without physical manifestations of an essential fatty acid deficiency.[16] Traditionally an essential fatty acid deficiency has been defined as a triene:tetraene ratio of greater than 0.2.

In a retrospective study of 214 neonates by Sanchez and colleagues[51] and a randomized controlled pilot study of 28 subjects by Rollins and colleagues,[40] lipid sparing appeared to prevent and slow down the onset of cholestasis. By contrast, in a much smaller retrospective review by Nehra and colleagues,[52] neonates with gastrointestinal disorders who received 1 g/kg/d of SO had a similar incidence of cholestasis when compared with neonates who received 2 to 3 g/kg/d of SO. Of note, there was a trend toward an increased rate of change in direct bilirubin in the 2 to 3 g/kg/d group compared with the 1 g/kg/d group, which did not reach statistical significance ($P = .05$).

All published studies investigating the efficacy and safety of SO sparing (1 vs 2–3 g/kg/d) for cholestasis prevention or treatment, with the exception of one small, randomized controlled pilot trial by Rollins and colleagues,[40] are single-center retrospective or uncontrolled prospective investigations.[16,51–53] As a result, methodological issues in study design and confounding variables, specifically advances in neonatal and nutritional care, have led to conflicting results.[16,51–53]

Likewise, all FO studies have been performed at one institution and most have relied upon historical controls.[44–46] In a small randomized, controlled study of 19 neonates of less than 3 months of age, there was no difference in the incidence of cholestasis and maximum serum direct bilirubin concentrations between the FO and SO groups. Interestingly one subject in each group crossed over to the other study arm because of a serum direct hyperbilirubinemia. The study was stopped early because of the unexpected low incidence of PNALD and concerns for futility.[39]

One concern with lipid minimization is the decreased energy intake from fat and the risk for a deficiency of essential fatty acids. Postnatal growth restriction and necrotizing enterocolitis in the premature population are inversely related to gestational age and directly linked to poor neurodevelopment.[34] Neonates with congenital gastrointestinal disorders are also at risk for long-term suboptimal growth and neurodevelopment.[54] To compensate for decreased calories many clinicians increase glucose infusion rates, which may promote cholestasis and steatosis. Although most lipid-sparing studies with either FO or SO have not demonstrated an increase in growth failure, these studies are not designed to examine such an outcome. Studies on long-term growth and development are clearly lacking.[16,39,40,45,46,51] Advantages to mixed lipid emulsions such as SMOF® are that they contain omega-3 fatty acids, can be dosed at 2 to 3 g/kg/d, and may better facilitate growth (see **Table 1**).

With regard to a deficiency of essential fatty acids, it does not seem likely that neonates receiving 1 g/kg/d and upward of FO or SO will develop a biochemical deficiency of essential fatty acids as measured by a serum triene:tetraene ratio.[10,16,45,46] However, deficiencies of specific fatty acids with lipid sparing and even toxicities with FO and SO may be possible, and may have unknown short-term and long-term consequences.[11]

Neonates, such as VLBWs and neonates with congenital gastrointestinal disorders who develop SBS, may possibly reap the most benefit from the potential hepatoprotective properties of lipid sparing or alternative lipid emulsions. However, one must also remember that these same infants are also at very high risk for nutritional deficiencies and cognitive delays.[16,34,41] As a result, it remains unclear if the possible benefit of lipid sparing (PNALD prevention and treatment) outweighs the possible risks (poor growth and neurodevelopment) in these high-risk groups. While some risk factors that predict clear and definitive intestinal failure and advanced PNALD are present at birth, many risk factors do not unfold until later in the patient's hospital course, making it difficult for clinicians to determine when to initiate FO or SO dose reduction (see **Box 2**).[1,2,37,41,55] Complicating this dilemma even further, the required duration for these therapies is unknown.[45]

In summary, direct comparisons of FO versus SO and 1 g/kg/d versus 3 g/kg/d of SO are complicated by the following: (1) published lipid-sparing studies have targeted different populations; (2) primary outcomes are different (cholestasis prevention vs treatment); (3) investigations have used different doses and durations; and (4) issues with trial design and sample size.[16,39,40,44–46,51–53,56] Considering the mounting evidence that FO may prevent or delay the need for transplant, it may be unethical to conduct a randomized controlled trial comparing FO with SO at 1 g/kg/d in children with advanced PNALD who are at high risk for liver failure or who have liver failure.[1,35,44–46] Considering the importance of PNALD prevention, it would behoove the research community to initiate well-powered, randomized, multisite, long-term studies, with or without a factorial design, to determine whether lipid sparing (FO vs SO, each dosed at 1 g/kg/d, and/or 1 g/kg/d vs 3 g/kg/d of SO) safely prevents cholestasis.

Lipids, Phytosterols, and PNALD

Understanding the reasons why FO, SO dose reduction, and mixed lipid emulsions may modify the incidence and progression of PNALD could provide important clues to the etiology of this disease. Such clues may uncover targets for future preventive strategies and therapeutics for PNALD. All 3 lipid strategies reduce the liver's exposure to phytosterols, which are known to interfere with bile acid transport, resulting in biliary sludge: the hallmark of pediatric PNALD (**Fig. 3**).[43,57–60] Phytosterols are found in vegetable foods and include campesterol, stigmasterol, and sitosterol. SO is made up of 43% cholesterol and 57% phytosterols. FO, by comparison, is made up of cholesterol only.[61] There is linear correlation between PN duration and increasing concentrations of serum phytosterols.[61] SO dose reduction and FO have been associated with decreased serum phytosterols.[62]

Approximately 5% to 10% of orally ingested phytosterols are absorbed by the intestine while 90% to 95% are excreted in the feces by the enterocyte apical ABCG5/G8 transporter. However, intravenous fatty acids bypass this transporter and rely on the canicular ABCG5/G8 transporter in the hepatocyte to secrete phytosterols into the bile. Sitosterol inhibits cholesterol 7α-hydroxylase, the rate-limiting step that converts cholesterol into bile acids, which plays an important role in lipid metabolism.[63] Moreover, stigmasterol antagonizes bile acid nuclear receptors, liver X receptor (LXR) and farnesoid X receptor (FXR). FXR protects the liver from hepatotoxic bile acids by reducing bile acid import via (1) suppression of the bile acid cotransporter (NTCP, SLC10A1), (2) reduction of bile acid synthesis by suppressing CYP7A1, and (3) enhancing bile acid efflux resulting from upregulation of the bile salt export pump (BSEP) ABC11 and organic solute transporter (see **Fig. 3**). In animal models, FXR knockouts develop liver injury, whereas treatment with FXR agonists protect against the development of cholestasis.[64] In cell lines, stigmasterol antagonizes BSEP.[65] Moreover, mice infused with PN and FO exhibited less liver injury in comparison with those infused with PN and SO. When stigmasterol was added to FO, these animals developed cholestasis.[43] Lastly, BSEP is developmentally regulated and is not

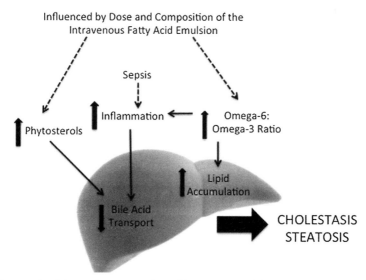

Fig. 3. Proposed etiology of parenteral nutrition–associated liver disease.

expressed or completely functional in the neonatal period, placing preterm neonates at high risk for PNALD.[66]

Lipids, Inflammation, Oxidant Injury, and PNALD

Bile acid transport is regulated not only by phytosterols but also inflammation (see **Fig. 3**). Critically ill neonates are at high risk for systemic inflammation, specifically bloodstream infections. The high mortality associated with long-term PN stems not only from liver failure but also CLABSIs, which can result in multiorgan failure and death.[2] Ninety percent of patients with intestinal resections develop cholestasis after sepsis, and serum direct bilirubins increase considerably after sepsis.[55] Lipopolysaccharides and cytokines alter the expression of specific bile acid transporters (BSEP and NTCP), decreasing bile flow.[67,68] When liver macrophages were stimulated with either stigmasterol, lipopolysaccharide, or placebo, cells subjected to stigmasterol or lipopolysaccharide showed increased transcription of interleukin-6 (IL-6) and tumor necrosis factor α (TNF-α).[43]

In a large meta-analysis, lipid products that contained FO or higher concentrations of omega-3 fatty acids were associated with a 25% reduction in infections (relative risk 0.75, 95% confidence interval 0.56–1.00). This finding may be the result of the immunomodulatory properties of omega-3 fatty acids and antioxidants in these preparations or chance.[19] SO is composed mainly of omega-6 fatty acids, which produce a cascade of proinflammatory bioactive compounds, and contains a small concentration of the antioxidant vitamin E. FO contains mainly anti-inflammatory omega-3 fatty acids and a higher concentration of vitamin E (see **Table 1**). Lipid emulsions that provide a more appropriate omega-6:omega-3 fatty acid ratio and contain EPA and DHA have been shown to decrease inflammatory mediators such as TNF-α, nuclear factor $\kappa\beta$, and IL-6, and increase proresolving lipid mediators, such as resolvins and protectins.[57,58] In neonates and animals, FO and mixed emulsions increase the concentrations of vitamins E and A and reduce lipid peroxidation, as measured by F2-isoprostane and total antioxidant potential.[47,49,50,57,58,69]

High omega-6:omega-3 fatty acid ratios also affect lipid metabolism by regulating peroxisome proliferator-activated receptor (PPAR) and sterol regulatory element binding proteins (SREBPs).[57,70,71] PPAR regulates fatty acid storage, whereas SREBPs are involved in cholesterol synthesis and fatty acid uptake. As fat accumulates in hepatic cells, phagocytic dysfunction and impaired endotoxin clearance occurs, resulting in hepatic injury. In fact, when rodents were provided with a high-carbohydrate, high-fat diet, supplementation with EPA resulted in improved insulin sensitivity, increased lipolysis, and decreased TNF-α and PPAR compared with animals who received a similar diet without EPA.[72]

LXR, which is regulated by phytosterols and inflammatory products, reduces production of apolipoprotein E, resulting in impaired clearance of chylomicrons and low-density lipoproteins.[73] In animal models, FXR agonists have been shown to be hepatoprotective by decreasing apolipoprotein CIII, which inhibits hepatic uptake of lipid-rich particles.[74] As a result, a lipid emulsion with a high omega-6:omega-3 fatty acid ratio may alter lipid trafficking, thereby promoting steatosis, yet another histologic feature of PNALD (see **Fig. 3**).

COST OF PN COMPLICATIONS

Considering that evidence-based and cost-effective medicine is essential to neonatal practice, clinicians must remember that PN can come with a significant price. For example, it is unknown whether the potential nutritional benefit of a short course of

PN for a low birth weight neonate (birth weight <2 kg) outweighs the daily cost of PN, which is approximately US $500. In one study, a NICU feeding protocol decreased PN duration by approximately 5 days, in turn leading to a significant reduction in cost: approximately $385,000 in hospital savings in 1 year.[75]

PN is life-saving, but complications such as PNALD and CLABSIs cannot be ignored. Once end-stage liver disease develops, the only remaining life-saving measure is combined liver-intestinal transplant.[2] Indications for transplant, either intestine or combined liver-intestine, include not only advanced PNALD, but also a history of repeated CLABSIs, which can result in catheter removals and replacements and eventual loss of vascular access. Five-year post-transplant survival is 50% to 70%, and the cost of transplant is approximately $900,000 in the first year post-transplant and $375,000 each year thereafter.[2,45] After transplant, patients are still not free of complications–which include graft rejection and deadly infections and malignancies secondary to immunosuppresion. With respect to CLABSIs, it is estimated that more than 2 million nosocomial infections occur each year in the United States. Almost half of all deaths in the NICU after 2 weeks of life are attributed to nosocomial infections, many related to catheters, and increase the average NICU stay by a mean of 24 days.[76,77]

SUMMARY

PN has revolutionized neonatology. However, potential long-term complications such as PNALD and CLABSIs are life-threatening, pose an economic burden to society, and profoundly affect the quality of lives of patients and their families. Research and collaboration is warranted to: (1) optimize PN delivery and composition to more closely mimic placental nutrient supply and that of a healthy, breastfed term infant, (2) identify biomarkers that reflect PN intolerance that are clinically relevant and predict the early onset of adverse complications such as PNALD and CLABSIs, and (3) reduce the incidence of PNALD and CLABSIs by improving current practices and developing new preventive strategies and therapeutic modalities. Together, basic scientists and translational and clinical researchers, along with clinicians and families, can improve PN care to enhance the health of all children.

REFERENCES

1. Christensen RD, Henry E, Wiedmeier SE, et al. Identifying patients, on the first day of life, at high-risk of developing parenteral nutrition-associated liver disease. J Perinatol 2007;27(5):284–90.
2. Squires RH, Duggan C, Teitelbaum DH, et al. Natural history of pediatric intestinal failure: initial report from the pediatric intestinal failure consortium. J Pediatr 2012;161(4):723–8.
3. Arnold M. Is the incidence of gastroschisis rising in South Africa in accordance with international trends? A retrospective analysis at Pretoria Academic and Kalafong Hospitals, 1981-2001. S Afr J Surg 2004;42(3):86–8.
4. Poindexter BB, Langer JC, Dusick AM, et al. Early provision of parenteral amino acids in extremely low birth weight infants: relation to growth and neurodevelopmental outcome. J Pediatr 2006;148(3):300–5.
5. Sekabira J, Hadley GP. Gastroschisis: a third world perspective. Pediatr Surg Int 2009;25(4):327–9.
6. Stephens BE, Walden RV, Gargus RA, et al. First-week protein and energy intakes are associated with 18-month developmental outcomes in extremely low birth weight infants. Pediatrics 2009;123(5):1337–43.

7. Bradnock TJ, Marven S, Owen A, et al. Gastroschisis: one year outcomes from national cohort study. BMJ 2011;343:d6749.

8. Mills JA, Lin Y, Macnab YC, et al. Perinatal predictors of outcome in gastroschisis. J Perinatol 2010;30(12):809–13.

9. Nandivada P, Carlson SJ, Cowan E, et al. Role of parenteral lipid emulsions in the preterm infant. Early Hum Dev 2013;89(Suppl 2):S45–9.

10. Le HD, Meisel JA, de Meijer VE, et al. The essentiality of arachidonic acid and docosahexaenoic acid. Prostaglandins Leukot Essent Fatty Acids 2009;81(2–3): 165.

11. Robinson DT, Carlson SE, Murthy K, et al. Docosahexaenoic and arachidonic acid levels in extremely low birth weight infants with prolonged exposure to intravenous lipids. J Pediatr 2013;162(1):56–61.

12. Boden G. Effects of free fatty acids on gluconeogenesis and glycogenolysis. Life Sci 2003;72(9):977–88.

13. Hey E. Hyperglycaemia and the very preterm baby. Semin Fetal Neonatal Med 2005;10(4):377–87.

14. Beardsall K, Vanhaesebrouck S, Ogilvy-Stuart AL, et al. Prevalence and determinants of hyperglycemia in very low birth weight infants: cohort analyses of the NIRTURE study. J Pediatr 2010;157(5):715–9.e1–3.

15. Hays SP, Smith EO, Sunehag AL. Hyperglycemia is a risk factor for early death and morbidity in extremely low birth-weight infants. Pediatrics 2006;118(5):1811–8.

16. Cober MP, Killu G, Brattain A, et al. Intravenous fat emulsions reduction for patients with parenteral nutrition-associated liver disease. J Pediatr 2012;160(3): 421–7.

17. Venick RS, Calkins K. The impact of intravenous fish oil emulsions on pediatric intestinal failure-associated liver disease. Curr Opin Organ Transplant 2011; 16(3):306–11.

18. Simmer K, Rao SC. Early introduction of lipids to parenterally-fed preterm infants. Cochrane Database Syst Rev 2005;(2):CD005256.

19. Vlaardingerbroek H, Veldhorst MA, Spronk S, et al. Parenteral lipid administration to very-low-birth-weight infants—early introduction of lipids and use of new lipid emulsions: a systematic review and meta-analysis. Am J Clin Nutr 2012;96(2):255–68.

20. Vlaardingerbroek H, Vermeulen MJ, Rook D, et al. Safety and efficacy of early parenteral lipid and high-dose amino acid administration to very low birth weight infants. J Pediatr 2013;163(3):638–44.e1–5.

21. Beardsall K, Vanhaesebrouck S, Ogilvy-Stuart AL, et al. Early insulin therapy in very-low-birth-weight infants. N Engl J Med 2008;359(18):1873–84.

22. Chacko SK, Ordonez J, Sauer PJ, et al. Gluconeogenesis is not regulated by either glucose or insulin in extremely low birth weight infants receiving total parenteral nutrition. J Pediatr 2011;158(6):891–6.

23. Mahaveer A, Grime C, Morgan C. Increasing early protein intake is associated with a reduction in insulin-treated hyperglycemia in very preterm infants. Nutr Clin Pract 2012;27(3):399–405.

24. Thureen PJ, Melara D, Fennessey PV, et al. Effect of low versus high intravenous amino acid intake on very low birth weight infants in the early neonatal period. Pediatr Res 2003;53(1):24–32.

25. Blanco CL, Falck A, Green BK, et al. Metabolic responses to early and high protein supplementation in a randomized trial evaluating the prevention of hyperkalemia in extremely low birth weight infants. J Pediatr 2008;153(4): 535–40.

26. Dinerstein A, Nieto RM, Solana CL, et al. Early and aggressive nutritional strategy (parenteral and enteral) decreases postnatal growth failure in very low birth weight infants. J Perinatol 2006;26:436–42.

27. Hay WW Jr, Thureen PJ. Early postnatal administration of intravenous amino acids to preterm, extremely low birth weight infants. J Pediatr 2006;148(3): 291–4.

28. Blanco CL, Gong AK, Green BK, et al. Early changes in plasma amino acid concentrations during aggressive nutritional therapy in extremely low birth weight infants. J Pediatr 2011;158(4):543–8.e1.

29. Blanco CL, Gong AK, Schoolfield J, et al. Impact of early and high amino acid supplementation on ELBW infants at 2 years. J Pediatr Gastroenterol Nutr 2012; 54(5):601–7.

30. Gravari E, Radmacher PG, Adamkin DH, et al. Amino acid profiles and serial blood urea nitrogen levels in infants less than 1250 g receiving early parenteral nutrition. J Neonatal Perinatal Med 2012;5(2):149–53.

31. Poindexter BB, Ehrenkranz RA, Stoll BJ, et al. Effect of parenteral glutamine supplementation on plasma amino acid concentrations in extremely low-birth-weight infants. Am J Clin Nutr 2003;77(3):737–43.

32. Denne SC, Poindexter BB. Evidence supporting early nutritional support with parenteral amino acid infusion. Semin Perinatol 2007;31(2):56–60.

33. Dusick AM, Poindexter BB, Ehrenkranz RA, et al. Growth failure in the preterm infant: can we catch up? Semin Perinatol 2003;27(4):302–10.

34. Cole CR, Hansen NI, Higgins RD, et al. Very low birth weight preterm infants with surgical short bowel syndrome: incidence, morbidity and mortality, and growth outcomes at 18 to 22 months. Pediatrics 2008;122(3):e573–82.

35. Willis TC, Carter BA, Rogers SP, et al. High rates of mortality and morbidity occur in infants with parenteral nutrition–associated cholestasis. JPEN J Parenter Enteral Nutr 2010;34(1):32–7.

36. Fitzgibbons SC, Jones BA, Hull MA, et al. Relationship between biopsy-proven parenteral nutrition-associated liver fibrosis and biochemical cholestasis in children with short bowel syndrome. J Pediatr Surg 2010;45(1):95–9 [discussion: 99].

37. Javid PJ, Malone FR, Dick AA, et al. A contemporary analysis of parenteral nutrition–associated liver disease in surgical infants. J Pediatr Surg 2011;46(10): 1913–7.

38. Baird R, Eeson G, Safavi A, et al. Institutional practice and outcome variation in the management of congenital diaphragmatic hernia and gastroschisis in Canada: a report from the Canadian Pediatric Surgery Network. J Pediatr Surg 2011;46(5):801–7.

39. Nehra D, Fallon EM, Potemkin AK, et al. A comparison of 2 intravenous lipid emulsions: interim analysis of a randomized controlled trial. JPEN J Parenter Enteral Nutr 2013;1–9. http://dx.doi.org/10.1177/0148607113492549.

40. Rollins MD, Ward RM, Jackson WD, et al. Effect of decreased parenteral soybean lipid emulsion on hepatic function in infants at risk for parenteral nutrition-associated liver disease: a pilot study. J Pediatr Surg 2013;48(6):1348–56.

41. Robinson DT, Ehrenkranz RA. Parenteral nutrition-associated cholestasis in small for gestational age infants. J Pediatr 2008;152(1):59–62.

42. Grant D, Abu-Elmagd K, Reyes J, et al. 2003 report of the intestine transplant registry: a new era has dawned. Ann Surg 2005;241(4):607–13.

43. El Kasmi KC, Anderson AL, Devereaux MW, et al. Phytosterols promote liver injury and Kupffer cell activation in parenteral nutrition-associated liver disease. Sci Transl Med 2013;5(206):206ra137.

44. Premkumar MH, Carter BA, Hawthorne KM, et al. High rates of resolution of cholestasis in parenteral nutrition-associated liver disease with fish oil-based lipid emulsion monotherapy. J Pediatr 2013;162(4):793–8.
45. Calkins KL, Dunn JC, Shew SB, et al. Pediatric intestinal failure–associated liver disease is reversed with 6 months of intravenous fish oil. JPEN J Parenter Enteral Nutr 2013;1–11. http://dx.doi.org/10.1177/0148607113495416.
46. Gura KM, Lee S, Valim C, et al. Safety and efficacy of a fish-oil-based fat emulsion in the treatment of parenteral nutrition-associated liver disease. Pediatrics 2008;121(3):e678–86.
47. Goulet O, Antebi H, Wolf C, et al. A new intravenous fat emulsion containing soybean oil, medium-chain triglycerides, olive oil, and fish oil: a single-center, double-blind randomized study on efficacy and safety in pediatric patients receiving home parenteral nutrition. JPEN J Parenter Enteral Nutr 2010;34(5):485–95.
48. Koletzko B, Goulet O. Fish oil containing intravenous lipid emulsions in parenteral nutrition-associated cholestatic liver disease. Curr Opin Clin Nutr Metab Care 2010;13(3):321.
49. Skouroliakou M, Konstantinou D, Koutri K, et al. A double-blind, randomized clinical trial of the effect of ω-3 fatty acids on the oxidative stress of preterm neonates fed through parenteral nutrition. Eur J Clin Nutr 2010;64(9):940–7.
50. Tomsits E, Pataki M, Tölgyesi A, et al. Safety and efficacy of a lipid emulsion containing a mixture of soybean oil, medium-chain triglycerides, olive oil, and fish oil: a randomised, double-blind clinical trial in premature infants requiring parenteral nutrition. J Pediatr Gastroenterol Nutr 2010;51(4):514–21.
51. Sanchez SE, Braun LP, Mercer LD, et al. The effect of lipid restriction on the prevention of parenteral nutrition-associated cholestasis in surgical infants. J Pediatr Surg 2013;48(3):573–8.
52. Nehra D, Fallon EM, Carlson SJ, et al. Provision of a soy-based intravenous lipid emulsion at 1 g/kg/d does not prevent cholestasis in neonates. JPEN J Parenter Enteral Nutr 2013;37(4):498–505.
53. Rangel SJ, Calkins CM, Cowles RA, et al. Parenteral nutrition-associated cholestasis: an American Pediatric Surgical Association Outcomes and Clinical Trials Committee systematic review. J Pediatr Surg 2012;47(1):225–40.
54. South A, Marshall D, Bose C, et al. Growth and neurodevelopment at 16 to 24 months of age for infants born with gastroschisis. J Perinatol 2008;28(10):702–6.
55. Sondheimer JM, Asturias E, Cadnapaphornchai M. Infection and cholestasis in neonates with intestinal resection and long-term parenteral nutrition. J Pediatr Gastroenterol Nutr 1998;27(2):131–7.
56. Cowan E, Nandivada P, Puder M. Fish oil-based lipid emulsion in the treatment of parenteral nutrition-associated liver disease. Curr Opin Pediatr 2013;25(2): 193–200.
57. Kalish BT, Le HD, Gura KM, et al. A metabolomic analysis of two intravenous lipid emulsions in a murine model. PLoS One 2013;8(4):e59653.
58. Kalish BT, Le HD, Fitzgerald JM, et al. Intravenous fish oil lipid emulsion promotes a shift toward anti-inflammatory proresolving lipid mediators. Am J Physiol Gastrointest Liver Physiol 2013;305(11):G818–28.
59. Kurvinen A, Nissinen MJ, Gylling H, et al. Effects of long-term parenteral nutrition on serum lipids, plant sterols, cholesterol metabolism, and liver histology in pediatric intestinal failure. J Pediatr Gastroenterol Nutr 2011;53(4):440–6.
60. Bindl L, Lütjohann D, Buderus S, et al. High plasma levels of phytosterols in patients on parenteral nutrition: a marker of liver dysfunction. J Pediatr Gastroenterol Nutr 2000;31(3):313–6.

61. Forchielli ML, Bersani G, Tala S, et al. The spectrum of plant and animal sterols in different oil-derived intravenous emulsions. Lipids 2010;45(1):63–71.
62. Btaiche IF, Khalidi N. Parenteral nutrition-associated liver complications in children. Pharmacotherapy 2002;22(2):188–211.
63. Boberg KM, Stabursvik A, Bjorkhem I, et al. Dehydroxylation of a 7 beta-hydroxy-C27 plant sterol in rat liver. Biochim Biophys Acta 1989;1004(3):321–6.
64. Liu Y, Binz J, Numerick MJ, et al. Hepatoprotection by the farnesoid X receptor agonist GW4064 in rat models of intra- and extrahepatic cholestasis. J Clin Invest 2003;112(11):1678–87.
65. Carter BA, Taylor OA, Prendergast DR, et al. Stigmasterol, a soy lipid–derived phytosterol, is an antagonist of the bile acid nuclear receptor FXR. Pediatr Res 2007;62(3):301–6.
66. Tomer G, Ananthanarayanan M, Weymann A, et al. Differential developmental regulation of rat liver canalicular membrane transporters Bsep and Mrp2. Pediatr Res 2003;53(2):288–94.
67. Moseley RH, Wang W, Takeda H, et al. Effect of endotoxin on bile acid transport in rat liver: a potential model for sepsis-associated cholestasis. Am J Physiol 1996;271(1 Pt 1):G137–46.
68. Ghose R, Zimmerman TL, Thevananther S, et al. Endotoxin leads to rapid subcellular re-localization of hepatic RXRalpha: a novel mechanism for reduced hepatic gene expression in inflammation. Nucl Recept 2004;2(1):4.
69. Deshpande G, Simmer K, Deshmukh M, et al. Randomized trial of fish oil (SMOFlipid) and olive oil lipid (clinoleic) in very preterm neonates. J Pediatr Gastroenterol Nutr 2013. http://dx.doi.org/10.1097/mpg.0000000000000174.
70. Perez-Echarri N, Perez-Matute P, Marcos-Gomez B, et al. Down-regulation in muscle and liver lipogenic genes: EPA ethyl ester treatment in lean and overweight (high-fat-fed) rats. J Nutr Biochem 2009;20(9):705–14.
71. Takeuchi H, Kojima K, Sekine S, et al. Effect of dietary n-6/n-3 ratio on liver n-6/n-3 ratio and peroxisomal beta-oxidation activity in rats. J Oleo Sci 2008;57(12):649–57.
72. Perez-Matute P, Perez-Echarri N, Martinez JA, et al. Eicosapentaenoic acid actions on adiposity and insulin resistance in control and high-fat-fed rats: role of apoptosis, adiponectin and tumour necrosis factor-alpha. Br J Nutr 2007;97(2):389–98.
73. Mak PA, Laffitte BA, Desrumaux C, et al. Regulated expression of the apolipoprotein E/C-I/C-IV/C-II gene cluster in murine and human macrophages. A critical role for nuclear liver X receptors alpha and beta. J Biol Chem 2002;277(35):31900–8.
74. Claudel T, Inoue Y, Barbier O, et al. Farnesoid X receptor agonists suppress hepatic apolipoprotein CIII expression. Gastroenterology 2003;125(2):544–55.
75. Butler TJ, Szekely LJ, Grow JL. A standardized nutrition approach for very low birth weight neonates improves outcomes, reduces cost and is not associated with increased rates of necrotizing enterocolitis, sepsis or mortality. J Perinatol 2013;33(11):851–7.
76. Mahieu LM, De Muynck AO, Ieven MM, et al. Risk factors for central vascular catheter-associated bloodstream infections among patients in a neonatal intensive care unit. J Hosp Infect 2001;48(2):108–16.
77. Polin RA, Saiman L. Nosocomial infections in the neonatal intensive care unit. Neoreviews 2003;4(3):e81–9.

Micronutrient Requirements of High-Risk Infants

Steven A. Abrams, MD[a],*, Keli M. Hawthorne, MS, RD[a],
Jennifer L. Placencia, PharmD[b], Kimberly L. Dinh, PharmD[b]

KEYWORDS

- Micronutrients • Premature infants • Nutrient shortages • Intravenous nutrition
- Calcium

KEY POINTS

- Preterm infants have unique and high requirements for bone minerals, including calcium, phosphorus, and magnesium.
- Guidelines for intravenous administration of these minerals emphasize preventing serum abnormalities such as a low or high ionized calcium or total phosphorus.
- A substantial issue, not yet fully resolved, is the ongoing shortage of minerals for intravenous use, requiring complex decision making to achieve the best and safest use of these minerals in high-risk infants.

INTRODUCTION: NATURE OF THE PROBLEM
What Are the Critical Micronutrients to Be Considered and Why?

The term micronutrient, as used in the context of infant nutrition, refers generally to any vitamin or mineral that is required for tissue growth and development as well as cellular or tissue function. This review focuses on the primary bone minerals, along with iron and zinc (Zn). The discussion of iron is limited to consideration of intravenous (IV) protocols for use, and the discussion of Zn is primarily limited to the problem of Zn shortages.

Sources of Financial Support: This work is a publication of the US Department of Agriculture (USDA)/Agricultural Research Service (ARS) Children's Nutrition Research Center, Department of Pediatrics, Baylor College of Medicine, and Texas Children's Hospital, Houston, Texas. Contents of this publication do not necessarily reflect the views or policies of the USDA, nor does mention of trade names, commercial products, or organizations imply endorsement by the US government. Conflicts of Interest: None.
[a] US Department of Agriculture/Agriculture Research Service, Department of Pediatrics, Children's Nutrition Research Center, Texas Children's Hospital, Baylor College of Medicine, 1100 Bates Street, #7074, Houston, TX 77030, USA; [b] US Department of Agriculture/Agriculture Research Service, Department of Pediatrics, Children's Nutrition Research Center, Texas Children's Hospital, Baylor College of Medicine, 6621 Fannin Street WB1120, Houston, TX 77030, USA
* Corresponding author.
E-mail address: sabrams@bcm.edu

Populations to Be Evaluated

Although the need for these minerals encompasses many groups of high-risk infants, the focus in this article is on 2 groups in particular: infants with intestinal failure, especially those with problems related to anatomic or functional short gut syndrome, and those who are very low birth weight (VLBW), less than 1500 g at birth. Both oral and IV requirements and provision of these micronutrients are considered, but much of the focus is on IV requirements and dosing.

Organization

The bone minerals, calcium (Ca), magnesium (Mg), and phosphorus (P) are considered together, followed by aspects of parenteral requirements for Zn and iron. Included also is a discussion related to nutrient shortages, especially for IV mineral components.

BONE MINERALS: CA, MG, AND P
Ca

One of the most important reasons for providing IV nutrition to high-risk neonates is to provide the bone minerals consisting primarily of Ca, Mg, and P. These nutrients also serve important physiologic functions, which can be critical in the neonatal period. The tools for assessing bone mineral status in the first week of life are minimal and do not fully reflect physiologic functioning.

The most difficult mineral to assess is Ca. For decades, total serum Ca was measured, and some attempted to adjust values for serum albumin. This approach was limited in usefulness at best and led to overly aggressive therapy at times in small infants. More recently, direct measurement of ionized Ca (iCa) has become widely available and used to assess status, but this does not change the fundamental problem that there are few clear data regarding either optimal or safe ranges for iCa in high-risk newborns.

Clinically, it is apparent that very preterm infants tolerate a lower iCa than full-term infants. It is common for a VLBW infant to have an iCa of 0.8 mmol/L without symptoms, whereas a larger infant would likely have neurologic compromise from this level of iCa.

We initiate IV Ca in the first hours of life in high-risk neonates whenever they are being provided with total parenteral nutrition (TPN). At our institution, this group includes VLBW infants, those with abdominal wall or similar abdominal defects, those with major congenital heart disease, and those with congenital diaphragmatic hernia. We provide 1 mmol/100 mL of Ca as part of TPN in a premixed starter TPN solution, which is usually provided at 80 to 100 mL/kg/d. This solution is available throughout the evening at our neonatal intensive care unit (NICU). P (see later discussion) is begun by 24 hours of age, usually at a 1:1 M ratio with Ca. Stability for standard starter TPN is 30 days when stored at 2°C to 8°C. However, sterility is the limiting factor to remain compliant with US Pharmacopeia (USP)-797 standards. USP-797 recommends a 9-day beyond-use date for medium-risk level sterile products.

Advancing to an intake level of 1 mmol/100 mL of Ca is dependent on maintaining an appropriate iCa. Our target range is 0.8 to 1.45 mEq/L in VLBW infants and 1.0 to 1.45 mEq/L in larger infants. Our goal is to reach 1.75 mmol/L administered at a volume of 130 mL/kg/d. At times, we advance to 2.0 mmol/L as well.

We consider the algorithm shown in **Table 1** for management of hypercalcemia in the first week of life in high-risk infants, especially those less than 1000 g birth weight.

P

Serum P is a reasonably accurate marker in early life of P status. However, there are rapid changes that occur even in healthy infants in the first week of life. Initial levels are

Table 1 Management of hypercalcemia according to iCa level in high-risk infants	
iCa Level	**Strategy for Action**
1.30–1.45	Recheck in 24 h Ensure that P is being provided at a (molar) ratio of 1:1–1.3:1 No change in IV infusion of Ca
1.46–1.6	Recheck in 24 h Decrease Ca infusion by 20% Maintain P infusion if serum P is 4–8 mg/dL Increase P infusion if serum P is <4 mg/dL May decrease P infusion if serum P is >8 mg/dL
1.6–1.8	Recheck in 12 h Decrease Ca infusion by 50%–80% Same guidelines for P as for iCa of 1.46–1.6
>1.8	Recheck in 8–12 h Stop Ca infusion Same guidelines for P as for iCa of 1.46–1.6

often increased and then decline over time. It can be difficult related to IV nutrition to provide appropriate levels of P via TPN and monitor it in the first weeks of life.

Nonetheless, it has increasingly become common to provide P earlier than was practiced in the past to VLBW and other high-risk infants. We now routinely add P to TPN by 24 hours of life and often before that. This strategy is because of our experience that this is safe and the possibility that a high Ca/P ratio leads to hypercalcemia, which is difficult to manage, especially in infants less than 1000 g birth weight.

Our practice is to add 1 mmol/L of P in TPN by 24 hours of age to keep the Ca/P ratio at 1:1 on a molar basis or about 1.3:1 on an mg/mg basis. In the first days of life, it is more common to have a low serum P of less than 3 to 4 mmol/L than a high one of more than 8 to 9 mmol/L. In general, it is difficult or impossible to directly attribute physical findings or other outcomes directly to the level of serum P in infants receiving TPN. We discourage frequent manipulations of the Ca/P ratio in attempts to correct minor changes in the level, unless it is persistently low or high, with general guidelines as provided earlier related to Ca. We recommend monitoring serum P at 24 to 48 hours of life and then every 2 to 3 days until feeding is primarily enteral.

Mg

In the first week of life, neonatologists are challenged to manage IV Mg therapy in VLBW infants because of the prenatal use of IV Mg in many women in preterm labor. Commonly, only a short maternal prenatal course of Mg is given, with little effect on the infant's Mg status, even when delivery occurs shortly after the maternal therapy. Our routine is to provide 0.5 mEq/L of Mg in TPN provided to infants after the first hours of life. There is no evidence to support routinely assessing serum Mg in high-risk newborns, although it is common to do so when the mother has received more than 24 to 48 hours of IV Mg within a short time of delivery.

Serum Mg levels can be low (<1.6 mEq/mL) or high (>3.0 mEq/L) in high-risk neonates receiving TPN. In general, low Mg levels are associated with fluid restriction and limited Mg intake. A renal wasting disorder is uncommon. Increasing the Mg concentration over a few days usually resolves hypomagnesemia. Aggressive intervention including Mg boluses over 1 to 2 hours are mostly reserved for infants with serum Mg levels less than 1.2 mEq/L, although there are no evidence-based guidelines for this.

Concerns about hypermagnesemia are more common than hypomagnesemia. We are cautious about removing Mg from TPN unless the serum Mg level is greater than 3.9 mEq/L. This caution is because symptoms are generally uncommon at serum values of 3 to 4 mEq/L, and the risk of having it omitted from TPN for an extended period and hypomagnesemia are of concern. Others hold the Mg from the TPN whenever the level is greater than 2.9 mEq/L. Usually, if Mg is omitted from TPN, serum levels should be drawn at least every other day and it should be readded when the level is less than 3.0 to 3.5 mEq/L.

ENTERAL REQUIREMENTS: OVERVIEW

The need for bone minerals to achieve adequate bone mineralization is a critical issue in high-risk neonates. This category includes VLBW infants but also other high-risk groups such as infants with intestinal failure. The role of bone minerals in the neonatal period is largely after the transition to oral feeds to prevent bone loss, especially clinical rickets. This topic has been covered in a recent statement by the American Academy of Pediatrics (AAP).[1] Highlights of this statement with some additional comments are provided in this review.

Box 1 lists factors that put preterm infants at risk for rickets. Key points are the critical role of nutrient intake restriction, which can occur as a result of conditions such as bronchopulmonary dysplasia. Medication use can also be important, with steroid use over a long period being a critical factor.

It is generally accepted that the primary problem leading to rickets in preterm infants is inadequate Ca and P intake. Achieving the in utero accretion rate of Ca of about 120 mg/kg/d is challenging, as shown in **Table 2**. In the United States, use of high mineral–containing human milk fortifiers or specialized formulas is a key aspect of management (**Table 3**). Transitional formulas are generally used at or near the time of discharge.

The role of vitamin D in this process is a complex issue, which is beyond the scope of this review. However, as shown in **Tables 3** and **4**, vitamin D should be provided to these infants. There is no evidence to support routine assessment of serum 25-hydroxyvitamin D levels in otherwise healthy preterm infants or for routine high-dose vitamin D supplementation.

RECOMMENDATIONS FOR DIETARY INTAKE

There are differences amongst groups in recommendations for the enteral intake of the bone minerals (see **Table 4**). The AAP report[1] provides recommendations

Box 1
High-risk criteria for rickets in preterm infants
Born at less than 27 weeks' gestation
Birth weight less than 1000 g
Long-term parenteral nutrition (eg, >4–5 weeks)
Severe bronchopulmonary dysplasia with use of loop diuretics (eg, furosemide) and fluid restriction
Long-term steroid use
History of necrotizing enterocolitis
Failure to tolerate formulas or human milk fortifiers with high mineral content

Table 2
Approximate Ca balance in a typical infant receiving 120 kcal/kg/per day intake

	Ca Concentration (mg/dL)	Intake (mg/kg/d)	Absorption (%)	Total Absorption (mg/kg/d)	Approximate Retention (mg/kg/d)
Human milk[a]	25	38	60	25	15–20
Preterm formula or fortified human milk	145	220	50–60	120–130	100–120

[a] Human milk assumed to be 67 kcal/dL, and preterm formula and fortified human milk assumed to be 81 kcal/dL.

consistent with current usual practice in the United States. Recommendations from Europe generally endorse lower amounts of Ca and P and higher vitamin D intakes. The safety and role of high-dose vitamin D intake, especially in infants less than 1500 g is undetermined.

Iron

The use of IV iron is uncommon in otherwise healthy preterm infants. It is more commonly considered for infants who are expected to have minimal enteral nutrition for more than 6 weeks. Previous concerns about the risk of anaphylactic reaction to the carrier have been decreased because of newer forms of these products (**Table 5**).

Multiple formulations of parenteral iron exist. If an alternative product must be used because of a back order, close attention must be paid to the specific product when ordering and administering. The incorrect selection or substitution of 1 formulation for another may result in overdosing or underdosing or serious adverse reactions if the dose or administration process is not adjusted.

Protocols for administration of IV iron are not widely available. **Box 2**, shows our clinical protocol. Before administering IV iron, we always check serum ferritin levels. Although there are no fixed standards for an increased ferritin level, we do not usually administer IV iron if the ferritin level is markedly increased.

Parenteral iron can be administered IV or intramuscularly. Intramuscular iron dextran use in neonates may be associated with an increased incidence of gram-negative sepsis.

Table 3
Intakes of Ca, P, and vitamin D from various enteral nutrition feedings at 160 mL/kg/d used in the United States

	Unfortified Human Milk[a] (67 kcal/dL)	Fortified Human Milk[a] (81 kcal/dL)	Preterm Formula (81 kcal/dL)	Transitional Formula (74 kcal/dL)
Ca (mg/kg)	37	184–218	210–234	125–144
P (mg/kg)	21	102–125	107–130	74–80
Vitamin D (IU/d)[b]	2.4	283–379	290–468	125–127

[a] Human milk data based on mature human milk.
[b] Based on an infant weighing 1500 g.

SINGLETON HOSPITAL
STAFF LIBRARY

Table 4
Recommendations for enteral nutrition for VLBW infants

	Ca (mg/kg/d)	P (mg/kg/d)	Vitamin D (IU/d)
Tsang et al,[2] 2005	100–220	60–140	150–400[a]
Klein,[3] 2002	150–200	100–130	135–338[b]
Agostoni,[4] 2010[c]	120–140	65–90	800–1000
AAP Clinical Report[1]	150–220	75–140	200–400

[a] Text says "aim to deliver 400 IU/daily."
[b] 90–125 IU/kg (total amount shown is for 1.5-kg infant).
[c] Reflects European recommendations.

DRUG SHORTAGES IN THE UNITED STATES

According to data provided by the Drug Information Services at the University of Utah in 2010, an average of 117 new shortages had been identified annually since 2001 in the United States; however, the number of shortages has met a sharp increase in the past 3 years, with 211 new shortages in 2010 and a record 267 new shortages in 2011. Between January 1, 2012 and December 31, 2012, a total of 204 new drug shortages were identified, down from 267 in 2011. Although 2012 was the first time in 5 years that a decrease in new drug shortages was seen, the number of active and ongoing shortages was still at an all-time high with 299 active drug shortages as of December 31, 2012.[5]

Tables **6** and **7** describe the reasons that drug back orders have become a public health and patient care issue.

There are several factors that contribute to a national drug shortage. These factors can occur at any point along the supply chain, including sources of raw material, manufacturers, regulators, wholesalers or distributers, prime vendors, group purchasing organizations, and end-user health care systems. It is important to understand why each drug shortage occurs to effectively manage the shortage.

On July 9, 2012, in an attempt to remedy some of these causes, President Obama signed into law legislation that gave the US Food and Drug Administration (FDA) new authority to combat drug shortages as well as impose new requirements on manufacturers. The FDA Safety and Innovation Act established an early notification requirement for manufacturers of drugs that are life supporting, life sustaining, or treat a debilitating disease when it discontinues a product or experiences a production interruption.[7]

Table 5
Injectable iron formulations

Components	Test Dose Needed	Concerns
High-molecular-weight (HMW) iron dextran (Dexferrum, Lutipold Pharmaceuticals, Shirley, NY)	Yes	Black box warning: fatal anaphylactic reactions may occur Adverse event risk is reported to be higher with the HMW iron dextran formulation
Low-molecular-weight iron dextran (INFeD, Actavis, Inc., Parsippany, NJ)	Yes	Black box warning: fatal anaphylactic reactions may occur (risk lower than with HMW formulation)
Iron sucrose (Venofer, American Regent, Inc., Shirley, NY)	No	

Box 2
Sample protocol for iron dextran administration to TPN-dependent infants

Order anaphylaxis medications (diphenhydramine, hydrocortisone, and epinephrine) to bedside to be administered only per physician's orders; physician must be present during test dose administration

Day 1: test dose: 0.2 mg IV once over 5 minutes

Day 2 of test dose: give iron dextran 0.5 mg IV once over 5 minutes

Day 3 of test dose: give iron dextran 0.8 mg IV once over 5 minutes

Monitor blood pressure during and after administration

Then start: iron dextran 1 mg IV every Monday, Wednesday, and Friday

National Shortage of Ca

Ca gluconate and Ca chloride are the only Ca salts available in the United States for IV administration. Ca gluconate is the Ca salt of choice in most NICUs. It is compatible with TPN and has a lower potential for extravasations compared with Ca chloride. In early 2011, the FDA issued a drug shortage for Ca chloride as a result of suspended distribution and manufacturing delays from several manufacturers. A national shortage of Ca gluconate soon followed as a result of the increased demand for the only available IV Ca alternative. Selected parenteral Ca preparations are listed in **Table 8**. Using different manufacturers and vial sizes may temporarily alleviate the shortage until an increased drug supply is made available.

Table 6
Impact of drug shortages

Higher drug acquisition cost	Need to purchase more expensive therapeutic substitutions Purchasing back-ordered products from alternative suppliers who charge 10–1000 times the original price[6]
Increased personal costs	Additional labor is required to manage back orders: keeping close inventory counts and comparing with usage patterns, researching alternatives, collaborating with physicians about alternatives/guidelines for use, making operational changes for alternative products (changes in database, labeling, and dilutions), and educating pharmacy employees, prescribers, and nursing about changes
Safety issues	Worsened clinical outcomes: there may be no alternative agent available, causing delays in medication procedures/therapies, or the alternative agent may not be so effective or may have a worse side effect profile Medication errors: substitution of different concentrations, resulting in an overdose/underdose, use of alternative drug products with different dosing, dilutions, and administration practices increases the error potential (especially in emergent situations)
Lack of adherence to clinical trial protocols	A back order of a drug used in a clinical trial may result in delay in patient enrollment Deviation from a trial protocol may occur when alternative products are used; this may cause the results of the trial to be questioned when analyzed
Loss of trust between health care professionals	Shortages can occur with no warning, requiring pharmacies to make abrupt changes; this may give the impression that pharmacy is not keeping good track of their stock and cause loss of trust Shortages are frustrating for everyone involved

Table 7
Factors contributing to national drug shortages

Limited raw or bulk material	80% of raw materials used in pharmaceuticals originate from outside the United States.[6] Factors that can decrease the supply of the raw materials involve: political problems that disrupt trade, animal diseases contaminating the source of the raw product, environmental conditions limiting availability of drug product supplies, or raw materials being contaminated during the acquisition process
Regulatory issues	Manufacturing plants are monitored by the FDA to assess compliance with current good manufacturing practices. If a company is found to be noncompliant, correcting these issues is usually a lengthy and costly process, leading some companies to close a specific manufacturing facility, resulting in drug product shortages, especially if they are the sole producer
Voluntary recalls	Voluntary recalls are usually related to an isolated manufacturing problem, such as lack of assurance of safety of specific lots, and are usually temporary situations. These problems can be safety related (eg, inability to assure sterility, possible glass particulates) or technical issues (eg, labeling, packaging)
Change in product formulation	When products have to be reformulated because of regulations (eg, changing propellants in inhalers) or change in the raw product (eg, changing from pseudoephedrine to phenylephrine), a shortage usually results because of the transition time
Change in manufacturer	Sometimes companies take over production of products that were being made by other companies. A shortage may result because of the lag in start of production by the new company compared with the halting of production by the old company
Business decisions	Drug manufacturers are businesses and make decisions based on financial return. If the financial return of producing a medication decreases, a company may decide to stop production of that medication, causing an acute shortage
Moving production locations	Many manufacturers have numerous production plants across the country. Sometimes, the decision is made to move production of one product to another plant, which causes a delay in production and therefore, a temporary shortage
Inventory management strategies	Companies at various points of the supply chain use a just-in-time inventory management strategy. This strategy improves a business's return on investment by decreasing inventory on hand and the carrying costs associated with that inventory. One problem at any point along the supply chain can result in a short-term shortage. Rural hospitals that cannot borrow medications or that are far from their wholesaler are even more affected by these types of problems
Acute changes in usage patterns	Production of medications is usually based on sales from previous quarters or years. If there is an unexpected increase in demand for a product, the manufacturer depletes their stock sooner than anticipated. This situation can occur when usage spikes because of a new indication being approved or when new medication recommendations are made by governing organizations
Alternative sources of medications	The national back orders have caused an increase in the amount of alternative distributors. These are companies that obtain medications for the purpose of reselling them at a higher price to hospitals in need of the medication. Obtaining medications from these companies is also worrisome, because you cannot confirm that proper storage conditions were followed during the chain of custody Compounding pharmacies often try to produce the medications that are in short supply. However, medications from these companies may not meet standards for aseptic techniques or labeling requirements
Natural disasters	Hurricanes, floods, fires, and tornadoes can result in loss of raw ingredients used in medications or cause damage to manufacturing facilities, resulting in shortages. The effect of these shortages may be worsened because there is usually an increased need for medications after such events

Table 8 Selected parenteral Ca preparations			
Product	Manufacturer	Concentration (mg/mL)	Vial Sizes (mL)
Ca chloride	Hospira	100	10
	American Regent/Luitpold	100	10
	Amphastar Pharmaceuticals	100	10
Ca gluconate	American Regent/Luitpold	100	50
			100
	APP	100	10
			50
			100

If there is critically low or no supply, it may be necessary to convert from one Ca salt form to another form, even after using different manufacturers. Ca salts have a varying amount of elemental Ca per gram (**Table 9**). Close attention should be paid when ordering and dispensing different salt forms of Ca. Substitution of Ca chloride for Ca gluconate without proper dosage adjustment could result in a 3-fold overdose. In addition, special attention is required to safely administer Ca (**Table 10**).

iCa reacts with freely available phosphate ions in solution to form an insoluble dibasic Ca phosphate precipitate. Ca gluconate dissociates into free Ca ions at a lower degree than Ca chloride, minimizing the potential for forming precipitates with phosphate in TPN. This property favors the addition of Ca gluconate to TPN containing phosphate. In addition, numerous studies have reported Ca and phosphate limits along with established Ca and phosphate compatibility curves, validating Ca gluconate as the Ca salt form of choice in neonatal TPN.[9]

However, a recent study by Migaki and colleagues[10] provided compatibility information for Ca chloride and sodium phosphate in neonatal TPN containing the amino acid, TrophAmine (B. Braun Medical Inc., Bethlehem, PA). Solutions were visually tested for the presence of precipitation and the investigators determined that amino acid concentrations of 3% or greater were compatible with a maximum sodium phosphate concentration of 15 mmol/L and Ca chloride concentration of 12.5 mmol/L. Although these data are valuable, additional studies under different study conditions are warranted before Ca chloride is used in neonatal TPN containing phosphate, because microprecipitates, capable of intravascular embolism, may exist even if in-line filters are used and visual observations are conducted.[11]

The precipitation of Ca and phosphate in TPN has resulted in at least 2 patient deaths and 2 cases of respiratory distress.[12] Insoluble Ca phosphate is a life-threatening hazard and a substantial patient safety concern. Although substituting Ca chloride for Ca gluconate in phosphate-containing TPN is a strategy to manage a critical shortage, this practice should be strongly discouraged. Ca chloride may be considered an addition to TPN only if phosphate is not present in the same solution. If Ca gluconate is not available, Ca chloride could be used in TPN without phosphate, administering infusions of phosphate separately. This is a potential strategy to

Table 9 Parenteral Ca salts				
	Salt (g)	Elemental (mg)	Elemental (mmol)	Elemental (mEq)
Ca chloride	1	273	6.8	13.6
Ca gluconate	1	93	2.325	4.65

Table 10
Infusion guidelines for Ca chloride and Ca gluconate

Concentration	For IV infusion, dilute Ca gluconate in normal saline or dextrose 5% in water (D5W) to a usual maximum concentration of 20 mg/mL for Ca chloride and 50 mg/mL for Ca gluconate. Undiluted drug (100 mg/mL) should be reserved only for bolus doses during emergent situations
Site of administration	IV administration via a central or deep vein is preferred. The following routes of administration are not recommended because of a high risk of severe necrosis and sloughing: intramuscular, subcutaneous, and IV administration via scalp, small hand, or foot veins
Avoid rapid administration	Rapid administration may cause a decrease in blood pressure, cardiac syncope, or extravasation. For Ca chloride, do not exceed 100 mg/min, except in emergent situations. For Ca gluconate, do not exceed 50–100 mg/min, except in emergent situations, in which infusion should not exceed 200 mg/min
Avoid intermittent infusions for maintenance	Intermittent infusions, even over 1 h, are nonphysiologic, potentially harmful, and should not be the standard way to administer maintenance Ca to a neonate[8]

Data from Lexi-Comp Online, Pediatric and Neonatal Lexi-Drugs Online. Hudson (OH): Lexi-Comp; 2011.

minimize the risk of extravasation from infusing a continuous Ca infusion separate from the TPN, because this risk is significantly less with phosphate.

In addition to phosphate, there are several common neonatal medications that are incompatible with Ca when infused via Y-site administration (**Table 11**). Determining

Table 11
Y-site incompatibility of Ca gluconate and chloride with common neonatal medications (not all inclusive)

Ca Gluconate	Ca Chloride
Amphotericin B	Amphotericin B
Ampicillin[a]	Ampicillin[a]
Ceftriaxone	Cefazolin
Dexamethasone	Ceftazidime
Diazepam	Dexamethasone
Fluconazole[a]	Diazepam
Hydralazine[a]	Hydralazine[a]
Hydrocortisone[a]	Hydrocortisone
Indomethacin	Indomethacin
Methylprednisolone	Mg sulfate
Meropenem	Methylprednisolone
Pantoprazole[a]	Pantoprazole
Phenytoin	Phenytoin
Potassium phosphate[a]	Potassium phosphate[a]
Sodium bicarbonate	Sodium bicarbonate
Sodium phosphate[a]	Sodium phosphate[a]

[a] Variable compatibility information.
Data from Trissel LA. Handbook on injectable drugs. Bethesda (MD): American Society of Health-Systems Pharmacists; 2013.

compatibility is highly complex and requires thoughtful consideration for safe administration. It is important to refer to the appropriate references (eg, *Handbook on Injectable Drugs*[13]) to thoroughly evaluate specific drug properties such as concentration and manufacturer, before concomitantly infusing medications with Ca.

Potential incompatibility issues are often addressed when patients have limited line access, which is a relatively common occurrence in the neonatal population. For example, if Ca gluconate is not available, the patient requires 1 line access for TPN and lipids, 1 line access for a continuous infusion of Ca chloride, and possibly another line access for intermittent medications that are potentially incompatible with TPN, lipids, or Ca chloride. Education on drug compatibility should be reinforced with the bedside nurses who are unfamiliar with infusing the alternative Ca salt.

Implementing institutional-specific guidelines is a practical strategy to conserve supply. Several federal and professional organizations such as the American Society of Parenteral and Enteral Nutrition (ASPEN) have provided considerations in approaching the national shortage of Ca, providing a good starting point for the clinician.[14] A thoughtful and reasoned evaluation is necessary to apply the information in an appropriate manner, recognizing what is clinically acceptable based on institutional practice and patient population (**Table 12**).

If a limited supply of Ca gluconate is available, it may be prudent to reserve it for neonatal patients. Neonates require maintenance Ca for their developing bones, and providing Ca in TPN is ideal for critically ill patients who are dependent on TPN for their nutrition. Also, neonates often have limited line access, which makes infusing Ca chloride outside the TPN challenging. Decreasing the amount of Ca provided in the TPN may further extend the supply and minimize the number of vials required to compound TPN daily (**Table 13**). This strategy may be applicable in large neonatal units or

Table 12
Applying considerations for neonates to ASPEN recommendations for Ca during a national shortage

ASPEN Recommendations	Additional Considerations for Neonates
Monitor serum Ca concentrations (iCa preferred or total Ca levels with albumin) if Ca gluconate is removed from TPN	There is a relatively greater iCa concentration for any total Ca concentration in very premature infants because of lower total protein concentrations. If iCa is unavailable, the corrected free Ca should be estimated with serum Ca adjustment formulas using serum albumin level
Infuse Ca chloride as a separate infusion from TPN	Adding Ca chloride to TPN containing phosphate is discouraged because of a high risk of precipitation. As a result of possible extravasation, it may be desirable to add Ca chloride to the TPN. In this case, remove phosphate and administer as a separate infusion from TPN
Consider multielectrolyte solutions containing Ca to prepare TPN	Multielectrolyte additives (eg, Nutrilyte, American Regent, Inc., Shirley, NY) are indicated as a source of replacement electrolytes for the depleted adult patient and not intended for neonatal use
Consider premixed manufacturer-prepared TPN containing Ca	Commercially available premixed TPN (eg, Clinimix, Baxter International, Inc., Deerfield, IL) is not formulated to contain the appropriate types and concentrations of macronutrients and micronutrients required for neonates

Table 13 Example guidelines to conserve Ca and phosphorus in neonatal TPN		
	Ca and Phosphate Limits	Considerations or Exclusions
Infants <1500 g	1.5 mmol/100 mL	Exclude patients with rickets, severe fluid restriction, or evidence of increased alkaline phosphatase, and then may increase to 1.75–2 mmol/100 mL
Infants ≥1500 g	0.6 mmol/100 mL	Exclude patients with rickets, severe fluid restriction, or requiring dialysis
Infants receiving <60 mL/kg/d of TPN and at least 60 mL/kg/d of enteral feeds	Remove Ca and phosphate from TPN	Ca and phosphate can be removed in patients who are TPN dependent for extended periods at these low volumes of TPN and on feeds (eg, short gut syndrome). Remove Ca and phosphate if alkaline phosphatase level is <500–600 IU/L

institutions that are able to compound customized TPN solutions. Institutions that outsource the compounding of TPN solutions should collaborate with the company to determine the severity of the shortage and identify strategies to reserve the supply for critical neonates or explore other compounding companies with potentially more access to the drugs in short supply. A minimum amount of Ca required for growth should be provided, and close monitoring of serum Ca is required.

IV Ca chloride as a continuous or short intermittent infusion is needed for nonneonatal patients. If Ca chloride is also in low supply, it may also be necessary to determine an acceptable lower limit of serum Ca before IV Ca is provided. If patients can tolerate oral feeds, oral Ca should be provided (**Table 14**).

National Shortage of P

Potassium phosphate and sodium phosphate are the only 2 IV P products commercially available in the United States. If there is a national shortage, using different manufacturers or vial sizes may be required to extend the supply (**Table 15**).

When procuring product is not possible to maintain the current usage, a shortage plan should be used to conserve supply (**Table 16**).

Total sodium and potassium content should be evaluated when switching to different phosphate products (**Table 17**). For example, when sodium phosphate is being used

Table 14 Selected oral Ca products			
Ca Salt	Elemental Ca (mg/1 g of Salt)	Elemental Ca (mEq/1 g of Salt)	Commercially Available Formulations
Acetate	250	12.7	Capsule, solution, tablet
Carbonate	400	20	Capsule, suspension, tablet, chewable tablet, powder
Citrate	211	10.6	Capsule, granules, tablet
Lactate	130	6.5	Capsule, tablet
Phosphate (tribasic)	390	19.3	Caplet

Data from Lexi-Comp Online, Pediatric and Neonatal Lexi-Drugs Online. Hudson (OH): Lexi-Comp; 2011.

Table 15
Selected parenteral phosphate preparations

Product	Manufacturer	Concentration (mmol/mL)	Vial Sizes (mL)
Potassium phosphate	Hospira	3	15
	American Regent/Luitpold	3	5
			15
			50
Sodium phosphate	Hospira	3	15
	American Regent/Luitpold	3	5
			15
			50

Table 16
Applying considerations for neonates to ASPEN recommendations for P during a national shortage

ASPEN Recommendations	Additional Considerations for Neonates
Use an alternate salt	Use sodium phosphate when potassium phosphate is on shortage and vice versa. Consider the total mEq of sodium or potassium contribution from the phosphate salt
Consider oral phosphate	Enteral phosphate replacement products should be used when possible. If a commercially available phosphate solution is not available, it may be appropriate to compound a solution from sodium/potassium-phosphate powder for oral solution
Consider premixed manufacturer-prepared TPN containing phosphate	Commercially available premixed TPN (eg, Clinimix, Baxter International, Inc., Deerfield, IL) is not formulated to contain the appropriate types and concentrations of macronutrients and micronutrients required for neonates
Decrease the daily amount of phosphate added to TPN	Refer to the example Ca/phosphate guideline limitations in **Table 13**
Reserve phosphate for pediatric and neonatal patients	Depending on an institution's usage, IV phosphate may have to be restricted only for neonates who are dependent on TPN and cannot tolerate oral therapy. Nonneonatal patients could receive replacement therapy if serum P levels decline below a predetermined level (eg, ≤ 1.5 mg/dL)
Reserve phosphate for patients with a therapeutic medical need	Phosphate may also have to be reserved for patients requiring continuous renal replacement therapy or who have diabetic ketoacidosis

Data from ASPEN parenteral nutrition electrolyte shortage. Available at: http://www.nutritioncare.org/Professional_Resources/PN_Electrolyte_Shortage. Accessed November 19, 2013.

Table 17
Mineral content of potassium phosphate and sodium phosphate

	P (mmol/mL)	P (mg/mL)	Potassium (mEq/mL)	Sodium (mEq/mL)
Potassium phosphate	3	93	4.4	0
Sodium phosphate	3	93	0	4

Table 18
Example guidelines for oral Zn administration with AquADEKS (Yasoo Health, Inc., Raleigh, NC) (for infants on TPN who would be receiving supplemental Zn because of losses associated with an ostomy or functional/anatomic short gut who are tolerating ≥30 mL/kg/d of feeds)

Infants >1500 g	Start with 0.25 mL once daily and titrate up to see if patient can tolerate the oral medication
Infants 1500–3000 g	0.5 mL once daily
Infants 3 kg to 1 y old	0.5 mL twice daily or 1 mL daily if tolerating well

instead of potassium phosphate, consider increasing potassium chloride in TPN to provide maintenance potassium if the patient has normal renal function. Caution should be exercised with orders for IV phosphate. The units (millimoles or milligrams) and salt form (sodium or potassium) should be used to express the phosphate product and total requirement.

National Shortage of Zn

Zn sulfate and Zn chloride are the only Zn formulations available in the United States for IV administration and are each produced by only 1 manufacturer. In mid-2011, the FDA issued a drug shortage for both Zn sulfate and Zn chloride as a result of suspended distribution and manufacturing delays from their manufacturers. Premature neonates require high amounts of Zn (400 µg/kg/d) because of negligible body stores of Zn, increased catabolic state, low albumin binding, and increased losses in the urine.[15] In late 2013, the FDA temporarily allowed for importation of Zn from non-US sources; however, the amount and distribution of this supply is uncertain.

Typically, trace element products that are available in the United States do not contain enough Zn to provide maintenance requirements to this high-risk population. Therefore, pharmacies must add extra Zn in these patients' TPNs. Additional Zn supplementation is also provided to patients with severe gastrointestinal (GI) abnormalities or losses. If injectable Zn goes on back order and needs to be limited, the first strategy of rationing can be to stop providing the extra Zn in TPN to meet goal maintenance requirements to reserve it for patients with severe GI losses. If it needs to be restricted more, patients' Zn levels can be monitored and supplemented only if low (**Table 18**).

If even further restriction is required because of an extremely limited supply, Zn can be administered only to patients who show signs and symptoms of Zn deficiency, such as impaired wound healing, alopecia, growth failure, immunologic impairment, and dermatitis. AquADEKS (Yasoo Health, Inc., Raleigh, NC) is a multivitamin and mineral supplement that is designed to help increase absorption of fat-soluble vitamins A, D, E, and K and other micronutrients. It contains 5 mg elemental Zn/mL so it can be used as an alternative to injectable Zn when patients are able to take enteral medications. Oral Zn formulations can also be compounded from tablets or capsules.

SUMMARY

Mineral nutrition in high-risk and preterm infants poses numerous challenges in balancing these nutrients and providing a safe infusate. Limitations in the supply of some of these minerals remain an additional challenge in providing these crucial nutrients.

REFERENCES

1. Abrams SA. Committee on nutrition. Calcium and vitamin D requirements of enterally fed preterm infants. Pediatrics 2013;131(5):e1676–83.
2. Tsang RC, Uauy R, Koletzko B, et al. Nutrition of the preterm infant: scientific basic and practical guidelines. Cincinnati (OH): Digital Educational Publishing; 2005. p. 277–310.
3. Klein CJ. Nutrient requirements for preterm infant formulas. J Nutr 2002;132 (6 Suppl 1):1395S–577S.
4. Agostoni C, Buonocore G, Carnielli VP, et al. Enteral nutrient supply for preterm infants: commentary from the European Society of Paediatric Gastroenterology, Hepatology and Nutrition Committee on Nutrition. J Pediatr Gastroenterol Nutr 2010;50:85–91.
5. Fox E, Wheeler M. Drug shortages in the US: causes and what the FDA is doing to prevent new shortage. Access Medicine from McGraw-Hill. Available at: http://www.medscape.com/viewarticle/780328_2. Accessed December 1, 2013.
6. Ventola CL. The drug shortage crisis in the United States. P T 2011;36(11):740–2, 749–57.
7. Food and Drug Administration Safety and Innovation Act (FDASIA). Available at: http://www.fda.gov/RegulatoryInformation/Legislation/FederalFoodDrugandCos meticActFDCAct/SignificantAmendmentstotheFDCAct/FDASIA/. Accessed November 18, 2013.
8. Brown DR, Salsburey DJ. Short-term biochemical effects of parenteral calcium treatment of early-onset neonatal hypocalcemia. J Pediatr 1982;100(5):777–81.
9. Trissel LA. Trissel's calcium and phosphate compatibility in parenteral nutrition. Houston (TX): TriPharma Communications; 2001.
10. Migaki EA, Melhart BJ, Dewar CJ, et al. Calcium chloride and sodium phosphate in neonatal parenteral nutrition containing TrophAmine: precipitation studies and aluminum content. JPEN J Parenter Enteral Nutr 2012;36:470–5.
11. Driscoll DF, Newton DW, Bistrian BR. Potential hazards of precipitation associated with calcium chloride in parenteral nutrition admixtures: response to Migaki et al. JPEN J Parenter Enteral Nutr 2012;36:497–8.
12. Lumpkin MM, Burlington DH. FDA safety alert: hazards of precipitation associated with parenteral nutrition. Rockville (MD): Food and Drug Administration; 1994.
13. Trissel LA. Handbook on injectable drugs. Bethesda (MD): American Society of Health-Systems Pharmacists; 2013.
14. ASPEN parenteral nutrition electrolyte shortage. Available at: http://www.nutritioncare.org/Professional_Resources/PN_Electrolyte_Shortage. Accessed November 19, 2013.
15. Centers for Disease Control and Prevention (CDC). Notes from the field: zinc deficiency dermatitis in cholestatic extremely premature infants after a nationwide shortage of injectable zinc–Washington, DC, December 2012. MMWR Morb Mortal Wkly Rep 2013;62(7):136–7.

Fatty Acid Requirements in Preterm Infants and Their Role in Health and Disease

Camilia R. Martin, MD, MS[a,b,*]

KEYWORDS

- Long-chain polyunsaturated fatty acids • Docosahexaenoic acid • Arachidonic acid
- Eicosapentaenoic acid • Linoleic acid • Lipid emulsions

KEY POINTS

- There is selective uptake and transfer of free long-chain polyunsaturated fatty acids (LCPUFAs) from the maternal circulation to the developing fetus.
- LCPUFAs are critical for many biological processes, principally organogenesis (especially of the brain and retina) and regulating inflammation.
- Current nutritional practices are unable to meet the intrauterine fetal accretion rates of LCPUFAs in the early postnatal period for preterm infants.
- Inadequate postnatal delivery of LCPUFAs results in early, rapid deficits in critical fatty acids, notably docosahexaenoic acid and arachidonic acid.
- Altered postnatal LCPUFA levels and n-6/n-3 fatty acid ratios in the preterm infant are associated with chronic lung disease and late-onset sepsis.
- Current scientific literature, including both animal and human data, support the role of LCPUFA supplementation in preventing disease and optimizing health in the preterm infant.
- The optimal strategy to delivery LCPUFAs to preterm infants to emulate recommended fetal accretion rates, maintain birth levels of fatty acids and their relative ratios, prevent early deficits in fatty acid levels, and achieve clinical benefit without potential harm remains to be defined.

INTRODUCTION

Enhancing somatic growth through our knowledge of macronutrient requirements (carbohydrates, proteins, and fats) is only one aspect of fully extracting the potential of nutrition to optimize health in preterm infants. The composition and balance of

[a] NICU, Department of Neonatology, Beth Israel Deaconess Medical Center, Harvard Medical School, 330 Brookline Avenue, Rose-318, Boston, MA 02215, USA; [b] Division of Translational Research, Beth Israel Deaconess Medical Center, Harvard Medical School, 330 Brookline Avenue, Boston, MA 02215, USA
* NICU, Department of Neonatology, Beth Israel Deaconess Medical Center, Harvard Medical School, 330 Brookline Avenue, Rose-318, Boston, MA 02215.
E-mail address: cmartin1@bidmc.harvard.edu

Clin Perinatol 41 (2014) 363–382
http://dx.doi.org/10.1016/j.clp.2014.02.007
0095-5108/14/$ – see front matter © 2014 Elsevier Inc. All rights reserved.

the individual building blocks within the macronutrients (sugars, amino acids, and fatty acids) are equally essential to understand. These building blocks often serve as bioactive molecules regulating many biological processes, such as organ development, metabolic homeostasis, and immune responsiveness.

Provision of fats is part of a balanced nutritional diet that delivers high-energy content, enhances gluconeogenesis, and prevents essential fatty acid deficiency. A large percentage of dietary fats are in the forms of triglycerides: 3 fatty acids on a glycerol backbone. Enzymatic hydrolysis releases the fatty acids from the glycerol backbone, allowing for trafficking and incorporation of the fatty acids into cell membranes, their primary site of action.

There is an extensive and evolving scientific literature showing the pleiotropic effects of fatty acids in health and disease. However, this literature is considerably more expansive for the adult than for the neonate. Despite this situation, strong evidence exists to support the beneficial role of fatty acids in neonatal health, especially in the preterm infant, and the need for ongoing efforts to further understand their mechanisms of action and to identify best nutritional or therapeutic strategies for delivery.

PLACENTAL TRANSFER AND FETAL ACQUISITION OF LONG-CHAIN POLYUNSATURATED FATTY ACIDS

Placental Transfer of Long-Chain Polyunsaturated Fatty Acids

Long-chain polyunsaturated fatty acids (LCPUFAs) are critical for the development of the fetal brain and retina. The importance of fetal acquisition of these critical fatty acids is highlighted by the presence of specific mechanisms allowing for maternal and placental transfer of fatty acids to the developing fetus. Although placental mechanisms for transfer are necessary, the synthesis of LCPUFAs in the placenta is limited, as it is in the developing fetus; thus, the maternal circulation is still considered the major source of LCPUFAs.[1–3]

Two major pathways have been proposed to facilitate the transfer of fatty acids from the maternal circulation, across the placenta, to the developing fetus: passive diffusion and protein-mediated transport (**Fig. 1**).[1,4,5] Maternal lipoproteins, triglycerides and phospholipids, are converted by placental lipoprotein lipase and endothelial lipase to form nonesterified or free fatty acids. Maternally derived free fatty acids are then transported into the placenta by passive diffusion or via protein-mediated transport. Transport proteins essential for the latter pathway include fatty acid transport proteins (FATP) 1– 6, of which FATP-4 seems to be of particular significance, because expression of this protein is directly correlated with docosahexaenoic acid (DHA) content in cord blood phospholipids,[6] placental plasma membrane fatty acid binding protein, and fatty acid translocase/CD36 (FAT/CD36). Once in the placenta, additional fatty acid binding proteins carry the fatty acid to the fetal interface, where FATP and FAT/CD36 deliver the free fatty acid to the fetal circulation.

Unique to this environment is the selective update and accumulation of LCPUFAs in the placenta and the fetal circulation, a phenomenon termed biomagnification. Labeled carbon studies tracking the transfer of fatty acids from the maternal to fetal circulation have shown higher DHA (22:6 n-3) content in cord blood versus maternal plasma, again emphasizing the unique role of the placenta in selectively transferring sufficient quantities of LCPUFAs to support the needs of the developing fetus (**Fig. 2**).[2,7]

Fetal Acquisition of LCPUFAs

The delivery of LCPUFAs substantially increases during the third trimester, coinciding with continued organ development and rapid fetal growth. Fetal accretion is targeted

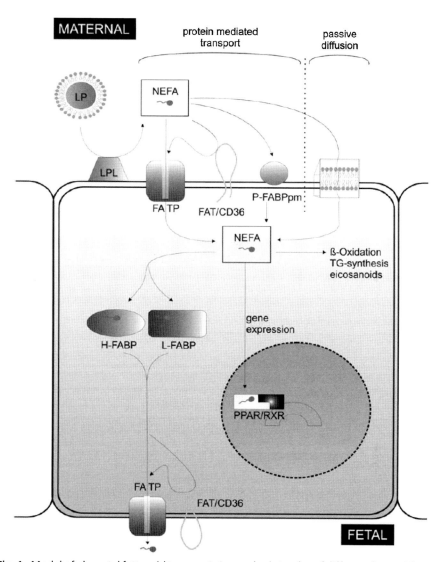

Fig. 1. Model of placental fatty acid transport. A complex interplay of different fatty acid transport proteins orchestrates fatty acid uptake by placental cells. Within the cell, NEFA are bound by different fatty acid binding proteins and have multiple functions like energy generation, TG, and eicosanoid synthesis, and activation of nuclear transcription factors like PPAR/RXR. FAT, fatty acid translocase; FATP, fatty acid transport protein; H-FABP, heart-fatty acid binding protein; L-FABP, liver-fatty acid binding protein; LP, lipoprotein; LPL, lipoprotein lipase; NEFA, nonesterified fatty acid; P-FABPpm, placental plasma membrane fatty acid binding protein; PPAR, peroxisome proliferator activated receptor; RXR, retinoid X receptor. (*Reprinted from* Hanebutt FL, Demmelmair H, Schiessl B, et al. Long-chain polyunsaturated fatty acid (LC-PUFA) transfer across the placenta. Clin Nutr 2008;27:688; with permission.)

to the brain, retina, and other lean tissues and organs. However, another important depot of fatty acids in the developing fetus is adipose tissue (**Fig. 3**). This reservoir is important to sustaining fatty acid requirements in organ development after delivery and throughout early infancy.[4] It is estimated that the delivery of long-chain fatty acids

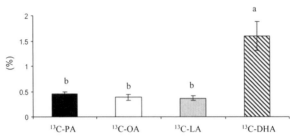

Fig. 2. Mean ratios between cord and maternal plasma area under the curve concentration of ^{13}C-fatty acids, expressed as percentages (n = 11). ^{13}C-PA, [^{13}C]palmitic acid; ^{13}C-OA, [^{13}C] oleic acid; ^{13}C-LA, [^{13}C]linoleic acid. (*Reprinted from* Gil-Sanchez A, Larque E, Demmelmair H, et al. Maternal-fetal in vivo transfer of [^{13}C]docosahexaenoic and other fatty acids across the human placenta 12 h after maternal oral intake. Am J Clin Nutr 2010;92:120; with permission.)

to support optimal fetal accretion is 43 mg/kg/d of DHA and 212 mg/k/d of arachidonic acid (20:4 n-6; AA) (**Table 1**).[8] In the preterm infant, this lack of accretion may have both short-term and long-term implications in predisposing to disease, as is discussed in the next section.

The most well-understood roles of LCPUFAs in the developing fetus are to support brain and retinal development. Approximately 55% of the brain comprises lipid, with the gray matter being 35% lipid, white matter 50% lipid, and myelin nearly 80% lipid.[9] LCPUFAs are a critical component of many of these lipid-based structural components, providing cell membrane structural integrity and fluidity within the phospholipid bilayer along with mediation of cell signaling pathways important in modulating the production of proteins that regulate neuronal differentiation and maturation, cell survival, and protection against oxidative stress.[2,10] Within the retina, DHA is concentrated in the outer segment of rod photoreceptors, playing an important role in differentiation and survival as well as the incorporation and function of the visual pigment rhodopsin.[10]

Much is discussed regarding the accretion of DHA in the fetal brain and retina; however, AA is the predominant fatty acid in the developing brain and retina until

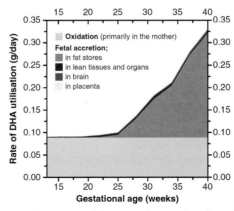

Fig. 3. Change in the rate of DHA use with stage of gestation. (*Reprinted from* Haggarty P. Fatty acid supply to the human fetus. Annu Rev Nutr 2010;30:239; with permission.)

Table 1
Estimates of the fatty acid accretion rate during the last trimester of pregnancy

	Per Day (mg/d)[a]	Per kg Body Weight Per Day (mg/kg/d)[b]
LA (18:2n-6)[c]	184	106
AA (20:4n-6)	368	212
LNA (18:3n-3)	7	4
DHA (22:6n-3)	75	43

[a] Adapted from Giorgieff and Innis [35]; the intrauterine estimate assumes tissue AA to be two-fold higher than LA [20,21]; the intrauterine estimate assumes that (1) DHA represents 90% of total n-3 fatty acids in all tissue except "other 0 tissue" [20,21], (2) the fatty acid composition of "other tissue" (20) is equal to that of skeletal muscle and that skeletal muscle contains 4.5% n-3 fatty acids [37], and (3) DHA represents 69% of total n-3 fatty acids in skeletal muscle [37].[8]
[b] Assumes weight between 25 and 41 weeks of gestation similar to Ref. [38].[8]
[c] Linoleic acid (LA), linolenic acid (LNA), arachidonic acid (AA), and docosahexaenoic acid (DHA).
    Reprinted from Lapillonne A, Jensen CL. Reevaluation of the DHA requirement for the premature infant. Prostaglandins Leukot Essent Fatty Acids 2009;81:145; with permission.

approximately 37 and 32 weeks of gestation, respectively (**Fig. 4**).[11] Thus, AA is likely critical to the biological development and function of these organs. Similar to DHA, AA plays important roles in cell division, differentiation, and cell signaling.[12] In addition, adequate AA is important in infant growth.[13,14]

Effect of Prematurity on Systemic Levels of LCPUFAs

Preterm delivery leads to an abrupt cessation in the maternal transfer of critical fatty acids. The early termination of fatty acid delivery coupled with the lack of adipose tissue stores make the preterm infant especially vulnerable to alterations in systemic fatty acids and fully dependent on postnatal nutritional replacement strategies while in the intensive care unit. The current parenteral and enteral nutritional management strategies fail to meet the LCPUFA fetal accretion requirements and thus do not allow preservation of levels that would have been otherwise seen if the infant had remained in utero for the final trimester of pregnancy.

Whether evaluating whole blood or plasma fatty acid levels, preterm infants show a decline in DHA and AA and a concomitant increase in linoleic acid (18:2 n-6; LA) levels (expressed as mol%) within the first postnatal week (**Fig. 5**).[15,16] In addition, the ratios

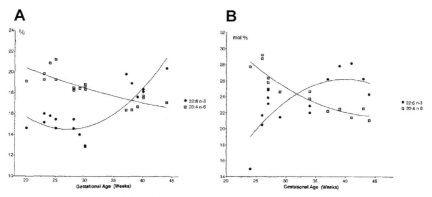

Fig. 4. DHA (22:6n-3) and AA (20:4n-6) as a percent of total fatty acids in forebrain (*A*) and retina (*B*). (*Adapted from* Martinez M. Tissue levels of polyunsaturated fatty acids during early human development. J Pediatr 1992;120:S131; with permission.)

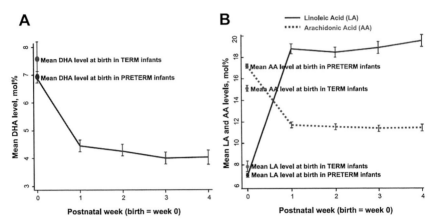

Fig. 5. (*A*) DHA levels in preterm infants decrease soon after birth and plateau by the first postnatal week. (*B*) LA levels in preterm infants increase soon after birth, and AA levels decrease soon after birth; both LA and AA plateau by the first postnatal week. (*From* Martin CR, Dasilva DA, Cluette-Brown JE, et al. Decreased postnatal docosahexaenoic and arachidonic acid blood levels in premature infants are associated with neonatal morbidities. J Pediatr 2011;159:746; with permission.)

of these fatty acids relative to each other are driven in the opposite direction of what is observed during the in utero period and at birth.

The rapid changes in fatty acid levels observed within the first postnatal week in preterm infants are principally driven by the current nutritional practices in the intensive care unit. Specifically, reliance on a parenteral lipid emulsion that is not tailored for the specific needs of the preterm infant and the delayed provision of enteral feedings that do not have sufficient fatty acid content (or delivery strategy) necessary to maintain LCPUFA birth levels lead to the observed profound alterations in systemic fatty acid levels.

Contribution of Parenteral Nutritional Practices to Altered Postnatal LCPUFA Levels

In the United States and much of North America, the principal lipid emulsion used for early delivery of fats to preterm infants is IntraLipid (20%, Fresenius Kabi/Baxter, Bad Homburg, Germany). Compared with the other available lipid emulsions (**Table 2**),[17] IntraLipid is 100% soybean oil, thus providing large amounts of LA but little to no DHA and AA. This lipid emulsion, approved by the US Food and Drug Administration (FDA) in 1972, was originally developed for use in the adult population. However, this product was subsequently applied to the neonatal and pediatric population, especially because no alternative has been approved for use in these specialized populations. Although provision of IntraLipid and thus the essential fatty acids LA and α linolenic acid (18:3 n-3) may be sufficient for adults dependent on parenteral nutrition, the provision alone of essential fatty acids is not adequate for the preterm population. The rationale for providing essential fatty acids alone relies on the presumption that the metabolic conversion of these fatty acids to downstream LCPUFAs is intact (**Fig. 6**).[18] Although not fully elucidated, it remains controversial whether desaturase and elongase activities are sufficient in the preterm infant to efficiently metabolize the precursor essential fatty acids to downstream LCPUFAs at a rate that meets their overall LCPUFA requirements.[19–21] In addition, it is not known how the unique metabolic state of the critically ill preterm infant affects overall fatty acid requirements. Regardless, it is self-evident that the provision of IntraLipid in the preterm infant is insufficient to maintain levels of LCPUFAs that emulate the patterns observed during the third trimester of pregnancy and at birth.

Contribution of Enteral Nutritional Practices to Altered Postnatal LCPUFA Levels

Not uncommonly, the preterm infant is provided with enteral feedings in a slow step-wise manner, such that the time to full enteral feedings to meet total energy requirements does not occur until, on average, the second postnatal week.[16] Thus, the enteral approach to administering fatty acids is unlikely to prevent the changes in systemic fatty acid levels that occur within the first postnatal week.[22] LCPUFAs are present in breast milk, but there is tremendous interindividual and intraindividual variation in mother's own milk and reduced levels in donor milk; thus, the levels that are present in human milk are unlikely to meet the total requirements of the preterm infant.[23,24] In the United States, preterm formulas have been supplemented with DHA and AA since 2002, but the current levels are not sufficient to prevent the early postnatal decline in these fatty acid levels. Furthermore, the bioavailability of these supplemental fatty acids is compromised by developmentally impaired lipolysis and absorption observed in preterm infants.[8]

HEALTH CONSEQUENCES OF ALTERED LCPUFA LEVELS IN PRETERM INFANTS

The changes in systemic fatty acid levels and n-6/n-3 ratios are directly linked to acute neonatal morbidities.[16] In a cohort of preterm infants less than 30 weeks of gestation, for every 1 mol% decline in whole blood DHA levels, there was a 2.5-fold increase in the odds of developing chronic lung disease (CLD). For every 1 mol% decline in AA, there was a 40% increase in the hazard ratio of developing late-onset sepsis. In addition, a positive change in the LA/DHA ratio was associated with an increase in the risk of both CLD and late-onset sepsis. These results are consistent with the biological role of LCPUFAs, especially DHA and AA, in regulating inflammation and immunity.

Although much has been described regarding the importance of DHA and AA in brain and retinal development, a direct causal link of low levels of these fatty acids to poor neurodevelopment has not been firmly established, especially given the many other competing risks for impaired neurodevelopment in the ill preterm infant. However, animal and human data on LCPUFA deprivation provide support for a critical role of LCPUFAs in neurodevelopment.

In weaning rats, 15 weeks of an n-3 deprivation diet resulted in a decrease in brain-derived neurotropin factor (BDNF) in the frontal cortex.[25] BDNF is an important signaling protein, which promotes Akt activation and, in turn, upregulates the CREB and mTOR pathways. Both CREB and mTOR are responsible for regulating gene expression and synthesis of proteins that are involved in neuroprotection, synaptic plasticity, actin organization, cell growth, and survival.[26,27] Nutritional modulation of BDNF is of clinical significance in the preterm infant. At birth, plasma BDNF levels in the preterm infant are lower than levels measured in term infants,[28] and the disparity in these levels may be exacerbated by the inadequate provision of n-3 fatty acids as a result of the current nutritional management strategies in the postnatal period of a preterm infant. Thus, the combination of low birth levels of BDNF and deprivation of critical LCPUFAs may place the preterm infant at risk for abnormal brain development.

In nonhuman primate models, plasma levels of fatty acids parallel the levels of these fatty acids in the brain.[29] As a result, the changes in whole blood and plasma levels of DHA and AA in the preterm infant previously described[15,16] are likely to result in changes in fatty acid composition in the developing preterm brain. Supportive of

Table 2
Commercially available intravenous fat emulsion products in the United States and outside the United States

| Product Name | Manufacturer/Distributor | Lipid Source | Concentrations of Selected FA, % by Weight | | | | n-6/n-3 Ratio | α-Tocopherol (mg/L) | Phytosterols (mg/L) |
			Linoleic	α-Linolenic	EPA	DHA			
IVFE available in United States									
Intralipid	Fresenius Kabi/Baxter	100% soybean oil	44–62	4–11	0	0	7:1	38	348 ± 33
Liposyn III	Hospira	100% soybean oil	54.5	8.3	0	0	7:1	NA	NA
IVFE available only outside the United States									
Intralipid	Fresenius Kabi	100% soybean oil	44–62	4–11	0	0	7:1	38	348 ± 33
Ivelip	Baxter Teva	100% soybean oil	52	8.5	0	0	7:1	NA	NA
Lipovenoes	Fresenius Kabi	100% soybean oil	54	8	0	0	7:1	NA	NA
Lipovenoes 10% PLR	Fresenius Kabi	100% soybean oil	54	8	0	0	7:1	NA	NA
Intralipos 10%	Mitsubishi Pharma Guangzhou/Tempo Green Cross Otsuka Pharmaceutical Group	100% soybean oil	53	5	0	0	7:1	NA	NA
Lipofundin-N	B. Braun	100% soybean oil	50	7	0	0	7:1	180 ± 40	NA

Soyacal	Grifols Alpha Therapeutics	100% soybean oil	46.4	8.8	0	0	7:1	NA	NA
Intrafat	Nihon	100% soybean oil	NA	NA	0	0	7:1	NA	NA
Structolipid 20%[b]	Fresenius Kabi	64% soybean oil 36% MCT	35	5	0	0	7:1	6.9	NA
Lipofundin MCT/LCT	B. Braun	50% soybean oil 50% MCT oil	27	4	0	0	7:1	85 ± 20	NA
Lipovenoes MCT	Fresenius Kabi	50% soybean oil 50% MCT oil	25.9	3.9	0	0	7:1	NA	NA
ClinOleic 20%	Baxter	20% soybean oil 80% olive oil	18.5	2	0	0	9:1	32	327 ± 8
Lipoplus	B. Braun	40% soybean oil, 50% MCT, 10% fish oil	25.7	3.4	3.7	2.5	2.7:1	190 ± 30	NA
SMOFlipid	Fresenius Kabi	30% soybean oil, 30% MCT, 25% olive oil, 15% fish oil	21.4	2.5	3.0	2.0	2.5:1	200	47.6
Omegaven	Fresenius Kabi	100% fish oil	4.4	1.8	19.2	12.1	1:8	150–296	0

Abbreviations: EPA, eicosapentaenoic acid; FA, fatty acid; IVFE, intravenous fat emulsion; MCT, medium-chain triglyceride; n-6/n-3 ratio, ratio of ω-6 fatty acids to ω-3 fatty acids; NA, not available.
[a] References 1, 10, 26, 37.[17]
[b] Fat source uses structured lipids.
Reprinted from Vanek VW, Seidner DL, Allen P, et al. ASPEN position paper: clinical role for alternative intravenous fat emulsions. Nutr Clin Pract 2012;27:156; with permission.

SINGLETON HOSPITAL STAFF LIBRARY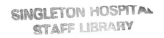

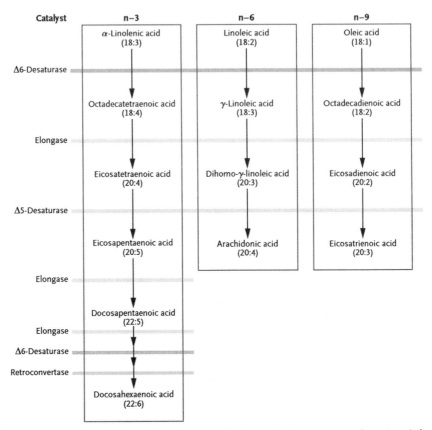

Fig. 6. An overview of the n-3, n-6, and n-9 biosynthetic pathways. (*Reprinted from* Freedman SD, Blanco PG, Zaman MM, et al. Association of cystic fibrosis with abnormalities in fatty acid metabolism. N Engl J Med 2004;350:562; with permission.)

this extrapolation are autopsy data that show abnormal DHA and AA content in the brain of preterm infants maintained on prolonged parenteral nutrition or high n-6/n-3 diets.[11]

EVIDENCE SUPPORTING THE ROLE OF LCPUFAS IN OPTIMIZING HEALTH IN PRETERM INFANTS

LCPUFAs play a critical role in cellular structure and function, including the regulation of membrane fluidity, cell signaling, and protein expression. It is through these intracellular pathways that LCPUFAs modulate immune and inflammatory responses as well as organogenesis (**Fig. 7**). Accruing animal studies and data from small human clinical trials support the role of LCPUFA supplementation to optimize the health of preterm infants. Examples are presented in the following sections for CLD, necrotizing enterocolitis (NEC), retinopathy of prematurity (ROP), and neurodevelopment.

CLD

As discussed previously, in a cohort study of preterm infants of less than 30 weeks of gestation, for every 1 mol% decline in DHA, there was a 2.5-fold increase in the odds of developing CLD.[16] By the first postnatal week, infants who developed CLD had

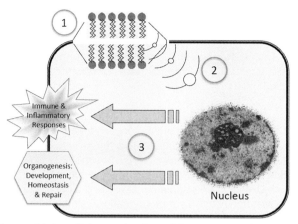

Fig. 7. Role of fatty acids in cellular mechanisms. (1) Formation of phospholipid bilayer of the cell membrane, (2) cell signaling, (3) regulation of protein expression responsible for immune and inflammatory responses and organogenesis.

lower mean whole blood DHA levels compared with infants who did not develop CLD (**Fig. 8**). The differences between these 2 groups persisted throughout the first post-natal month. Supporting these observational data is the reduction of CLD in breast milk–fed infants less than 1250 g whose mothers were supplemented with a high-DHA diet compared with infants whose mothers were not supplemented (34.5% vs 47%, respectively).[30] In addition, in a small clinical trial comparing delivery of IntraLi-pid versus SMOFlipid (15% fish oil) in preterm infants, the subgroup of infants less

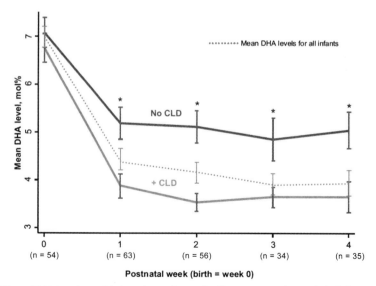

Fig. 8. Mean DHA levels are higher throughout the first postnatal month in infants without CLD compared with infants with CLD. *All *P* values <.02 comparing the mean DHA level in each postnatal week in infants with and without CLD. Bars represent standard error of the mean. (*Reprinted from* Martin CR, Dasilva DA, Cluette-Brown JE, et al. Decreased postnatal docosahexaenoic and arachidonic acid blood levels in premature infants are associated with neonatal morbidities. J Pediatr 2011;159:746; with permission.)

than 1500 g who received SMOFlipid were less likely to develop CLD.[31] Animal data provide further biological plausibility for the role of LCPUFAs in ameliorating neonatal lung injury. In a murine model of neonatal hyperoxia-induced lung injury, increased exposure to DHA, either through increased maternal content in dam milk or directly through oral administration to the mouse pups, ameliorated the expression of lung injury with reduction of inflammatory biomarkers[32,33] and improved alveolarization.[32]

NEC

In a rat model of NEC, the incidence of NEC was reduced with enteral supplementation of LCPUFAs, with the greatest reduction in the groups supplemented with DHA (50% reduction) or both DHA and AA (30% reduction).[34] Mechanisms proposed include a decrease in platelet-activating factor messenger RNA (mRNA) expression in response to both DHA and AA supplementation and a decrease in toll-like receptor 4 (TLR4) mRNA expression with AA supplementation. Clinical trials of LCPUFA supplementation in preterm infants have not shown a reduction in NEC. However, the few trials of LCPUFA supplementation in preterm infants were not designed to study NEC as a primary aim nor were they adequately powered to look at NEC even as a secondary outcome. The best supporting evidence for the potential role of LCPUFAs in preventing NEC comes from the scientific literature in inflammatory bowel disease, an intestinal disease process that may share similar mechanisms with NEC.[35,36] The current scientific literature supports an immunomodulatory role of LCPUFAs at the level of the enterocyte, including inhibition of TLR4 expression; downregulation of nuclear factor B (NF-B) signaling of inflammatory biomarkers through interaction with the nuclear receptor, peroxisome proliferator activated receptor (PPAR), or through the production of antiinflammatory terminal metabolites of DHA, such as the resolvin D series; and, through modulation of other fatty acid–derived proinflammatory cytokines such as eicosanoids (**Fig. 9**).[35]

ROP

In preterm infants of less than 32 weeks of gestation and less than 1250 g given either a standard lipid emulsion without fish oil or a standard lipid emulsion blended with 100% fish oil (Omegaven), the infants receiving fish oil had a trend toward a reduced incidence of ROP requiring laser therapy.[37] Supporting this clinical finding are results from a murine model of ROP. Pups born to mothers with an n-3–dominant diet versus an n-6–dominant diet showed less retinal vaso-obliteration and neovascularization secondary to hyperoxia exposure.[38] In addition, the same protective effect against retinal injury with hyperoxia was found in pups in the n-6–dominant diet group when concurrently provided resolvin D1, resolvin E1 or neuroprotectin D1, all terminal antiinflammatory, bioactive metabolites of the n-3 fatty acids, DHA and eicosapentaenoic acid (EPA). The protective effect of the n-3 fatty acid diet seems to be partially mediated through a downregulation of tumor necrosis factor mRNA expression in the retina.

Neurodevelopment

Overall, the data for long-term neurodevelopmental benefits of LCPUFA supplementation in preterm infants are mixed.[39] Some of the potential reasons for this finding are discussed in more detail later and include considerations such as dosing, timing of delivery, and bioavailability with enteral consumption. However, intriguing data are accumulating regarding the role of LCPUFAs in upregulating signaling pathways important for brain development, reducing lipopolysaccharide (LPS)-induced neuronal injury and attenuating the sequelae of traumatic brain injury. It was previously discussed that, compared with term newborns, preterm infants have lower levels of

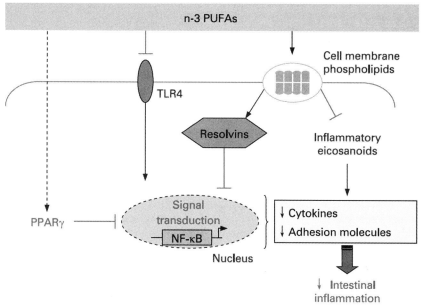

Fig. 9. Mechanisms of action of n-3 polyunsaturated fatty acids (PUFAs) in intestinal inflammation. The n-3 PUFAs activate peroxisome proliferator activated receptor c (PPARc), which inhibits the NF-κB signaling pathway. The effects of n-3 PUFAs may also inhibit TLR4. The n-3 PUFAs could also modulate fatty acid composition in cell membrane phospholipids, leading to a decrease of inflammatory eicosanoids derived from AA and to an increased production of antiinflammatory compounds such as resolvins. These regulatory pathways lead to decreased generation of proinflammatory cytokines and decreased expression of adhesion molecules, resulting in an inhibition of intestinal inflammation. (*Reprinted from* Marion-Letellier R, Dechelotte P, Iacucci M, et al. Dietary modulation of peroxisome proliferator-activated receptor gamma. Gut 2009;58:588; with permission.)

BDNF,[28] which can be further compromised with n-3 fatty acid deprivation.[25] The investigators of the latter study also reported that BDNF protein levels can be restored with DHA supplementation. Adequate levels of BDNF allow for downstream activation of the Akt, CREB, and mTOR pathways, all critical pathways in the regulation of proteins involved in brain organogenesis, homeostasis, and repair.

Neonatal sepsis is an independent risk factor for poor neurocognitive outcomes.[40] It is hypothesized that systemic inflammation leads to microglial activation and subsequent oxidative injury and cell death. In vitro studies of cultured LPS-activated glial cells show a DHA dose-dependent effect in reducing oxidative injury and attenuating the production of proinflammatory biomarkers.[41] Furthermore, in a neonatal murine model of cerebral hypoxic ischemic injury, provision of DHA after the brain insult decreased the total infarction volume and thus brain injury.[42] Although, not specifically evaluated, it was speculated that the protective effect of DHA was imparted by reducing oxidative injury and subsequent cell death.

CHALLENGES IN DELIVERING LCPUFAS TO PRETERM INFANTS

Nutritional delivery to the preterm infant largely consists of 2 phases: the parenteral phase, in which much of the nutritional content is delivered intravenously, and the enteral phase, in which most of the nutritional intake is given through the gut. As a result, delivering LCPUFAs to meet fetal accretion rates and to prevent the early alterations in postnatal changes in fatty acid levels must consider both phases.

Parenteral

As described earlier, the commonly used lipid emulsion in the United States, IntraLipid, fails to meet the fatty acid requirements of the preterm infant. Other lipid emulsions are commercially available but have not received FDA approval. However, it is not clear that even these emulsions fully meet the specific needs of the preterm infant. Ideally, any lipid emulsion uniquely tailored for the preterm infant should meet intrauterine fetal accretion rates of critical LCPUFAs, which, in addition, would maintain birth levels of these fatty acids (ie, prevent the early decline of DHA and AA and minimize the increase in LA). Small trials comparing various lipid emulsions in the preterm population indicate that currently available preparations are unable to preserve critical LCPUFA levels and, furthermore, may lead to changes in other fatty acids, which may pose different risks.

Forty-eight preterm infants with birth weights between 500 g and 1249 g were randomized to receive a standard lipid emulsion (50:50 medium-chain triglyceride [MCT]/soybean oil) or a study lipid emulsion containing 10% fish oil, 50% MCT, and 40% soybean oil. Plasma phospholipid levels of AA, DHA, and EPA were determined at birth, postnatal day 7, and postnatal day 14 (**Fig. 10**).[43] Compared with the standard lipid

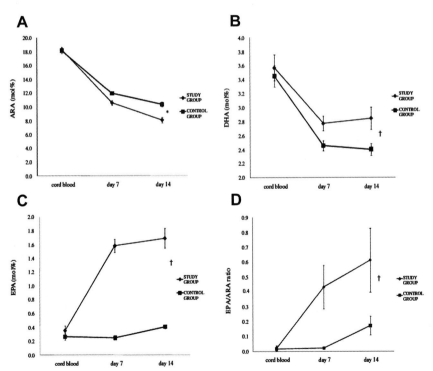

Fig. 10. (A) AA; (B) DHA; (C) EPA content, as mol%; and (D) EPA/AA ratio in plasma phospholipids (mean ± standard error of the mean) at day 0 (cord blood), day 7, and day 14. *$P = .02$. †$P<.01$. (*Reprinted from* D'Ascenzo R, D'Egidio S, Angelini L, et al. Parenteral nutrition of preterm infants with a lipid emulsion containing 10% fish oil: effect on plasma lipids and long-chain polyunsaturated fatty acids. J Pediatr 2011;159:36; with permission.)

emulsion group, receipt of the study lipid emulsion with 10% fish oil did not change the overall postnatal decline in DHA and AA levels. DHA plasma phospholipid levels were only slightly greater in the fish oil group compared with the standard lipid emulsion group, and AA levels decreased in the fish oil group versus the standard lipid group. There was a substantial, almost 5-fold increase in EPA (20:5 n-3) levels in the fish oil group versus standard lipid group.

Although other small clinical trials of lipid emulsions containing fish oil have been conducted, few have adequately described the changes in systemic fatty acid profiles with parenteral administration of fish oil. Considering the data described earlier, increasing the fish oil content of the lipid emulsion from 10% (Lipoplus) to 15% (SMO-Flipid) to 100% (Omegaven) may lead to more exaggerated fatty acid profiles compared with those described in the preceding paragraph. Thus, providing enriched DHA and EPA substantially increases DHA and EPA levels, but because of lower delivery of LA and substrate competition between n-3 and n-6 fatty acids, systemic levels of AA would decrease further. Supporting this premise are data from older, parenteral nutrition–dependent preterm infants who were switched from a predominantly soybean lipid emulsion to one containing a high concentration of fish oil.[44] Over time, plasma fatty acid patterns showed an 8-fold increase in DHA, a more than 20-fold increase in EPA, and a substantial decrease in LA and AA levels.

Although increasing levels of DHA may be clinically desirable, a concomitant increase in EPA may produce unknown but potential, adverse effects in the preterm population. Prolific literature on the role of n-3 fatty acids in adult cardiovascular health show biological effects of these fatty acids in inhibiting platelet-activating factor, decreasing platelet aggregation, and increasing bleeding time.[45] In addition, n-3 fatty acids reduce plasma triglyceride levels and the delivery of cholesterol to tissues. Unique to EPA is the decrease in natural killer cell activity and in T-lymphocyte function with increasing levels. All of these effects may be beneficial in an adult with cardiovascular disease; however, these effects may be problematic in the preterm infant, in whom there is a developmental bleeding diathesis and risk for intracranial hemorrhage, immune dysfunction, and a nutritional need for triglyceride and cholesterol production for organ development. The decrease in AA levels seen in parallel with enriched DHA/EPA delivery may be of concern given the critical functions that AA serves in brain and eye development as well as overall growth. Different lipid emulsions need to be developed and studied to meet the unique LCPUFA needs of the preterm infant. It is imperative to carefully quantify the changes in systemic fatty acid profiles with novel lipid emulsions and document potential side effects of the changing fatty acid profiles in addition to its potential clinical benefits.

Enteral

Despite the presence of LCPUFAs in human milk as well as DHA and AA supplementation in formulas, dietary provision of breast milk or formula fails to meet the fatty acid requirements in preterm infants[22] or fully attain the potential neurocognitive and visual benefits of fatty acid supplementation.[39] Although some clinical trials of LCPUFA supplementation have shown short-term benefits in neurocognitive outcomes and visual motor function, these benefits are not sustained nor shown consistently in all studies. The lack of a clear benefit of LCPUFA supplementation likely reflects inadequate LCPUFA timing and delivery rather than a failure of clinical benefit from the fatty acid itself. Many enteral supplementation studies have started the supplementation after the infant has begun on enteral feedings or after the infant has achieved a substantial daily intake by the enteral route, both of these time points well after the time when deficits in systemic DHA and AA levels have already occurred in the preterm infant.

Another factor complicating the enteral delivery of LCPUFAs is the ability of the preterm infant to hydrolyze dietary triglycerides to allow absorption of the resultant monoglycerides and free fatty acids. A measure of efficient fat hydrolysis and absorption is the coefficient of fat absorption (CFA), which is expressed as the fraction (percent) of the difference between total fat intake and total fecal fat losses over total fat intake. A perfect rate of hydrolysis and absorption is 100%, with normal values being greater than 90%. Thus, the higher the CFA value, the more efficient the hydrolysis and absorption. This value can be calculated for total fat as well as for individual fatty acids. Total CFA and specific fatty acid CFAs for DHA and AA all show values in the 70% to 80% range in preterm infants fed formula or pasteurized human milk.[46] The lower DHA and AA CFA values in infants fed formula and pasteurized human milk may be accounted for by developmental pancreatic insufficiency and decreased production of lipase as well as a reduction in bile acid pools. Preterm infants fed mother's own milk (nonpasteurized) show higher CFA levels, likely because of the presence of bile salt–stimulated lipase in the milk, which is absent in formula and degraded in pasteurized human milk.

Increasing the total content of DHA and AA in formulas to overcome the limitations in lipid hydrolysis and intestinal absorption may be of limited value. In a lipase-deficient murine model, enteral delivery of fats led to lipid-laden fat accumulation in the intestinal enterocytes and intestinal injury.[47] Thus, the effects of surpassing the capacity of the preterm infant's ability to hydrolyze and absorb dietary fatty acids are unknown but may be potentially harmful to the developing gut.

Enteral delivery of nutrients is preferred over parenteral administration. However, adequate delivery of enteral fatty acids that translates to improved systemic fatty acid profiles needs to consider and overcome the inadequacy of the current dosing of DHA and AA in formula and breast milk to meet the fatty acid requirements of the preterm infant. This necessity is especially important during the early postnatal period, when the relative decrease in lipase production and bile acid pools to efficiently hydrolyze and absorb enterally administered fatty acids is at play.

Maternal

Another potential route to increase LCPUFA levels in the preterm infant is through maternal strategies. An increase in the intake of maternal LCPUFAs can increase the breast milk content of LCPUFAs, allowing for more efficient delivery to the preterm infant. Although this strategy can lead to higher LCPUFA levels in the preterm infant and is important in maintaining LCPUFA levels during the enteral phase of nutrition,[48] it is unlikely that this strategy alone ameliorates the deficits in LCPUFA levels that become evident in the early postnatal period.

FUTURE DIRECTIONS

The premise that LCPUFAs are essential for neonatal health is validated given:

- The presence of specialized mechanisms to enhance placental transfer from the mother to the developing fetus
- Their biological roles in fetal development, ongoing organogenesis, and regulation of inflammation
- Accruing promising data supporting their immunomodulatory capabilities in ameliorating neonatal disease pathogenesis and optimizing normal development

However, before implementing new practices, either adopting new lipid emulsions or administering new enteral formulations, careful research needs to be conducted to understand the balance of what is required, for what therapeutic goal, and to minimize potential harm.

Questions and concepts that need to be thoroughly considered include:

- What is our therapeutic goal? Is it to fully emulate our current understanding of fetal accretion rates? Is it to provide doses that support maintenance requirements to maintain birth levels of fatty acids and ongoing development? Or is it to provide doses that target specific disease processes or inflammatory states?
- What are the target levels (whole blood, plasma, tissue, or even cellular) and fatty acid ratios that need to be attained to achieve the therapeutic goal? How are these target levels modified, given the acuity and metabolic state of the infant?
- What are the unique challenges with parenteral delivery of fatty acids versus enteral delivery? What is the ideal formulation, including the biochemical structure, that supports fatty acid hydrolysis, absorption, and incorporation into the target tissue?
- What are biochemical assays and clinical parameters that need to collected and evaluated to ensure the optimal balance between clinical benefit and potential harm?

SUMMARY

The preterm infant presents a unique challenge but an exciting opportunity to define the role of LCPUFAs in both maintenance of health and prevention of disease. Through understanding of basic mechanisms and the pathophysiologic consequences of altered fatty acid levels, the provision of critical fatty acids through parenteral or enteral routes can mitigate the risk of diseases such as CLD, nosocomial sepsis, NEC, ROP, and neurocognitive impairment. The challenge is to understand the changing nutritional and therapeutic goals along a developmental timeline with superimposed exposures to disease risks. The result is an effect on immunomodulatory functions, organ development, and neuroprotection. Diligent research efforts to further define fetal accretion requirements, mechanisms of intestinal fatty acid lipolysis and absorption, and fatty acid metabolism and tissue incorporation will provide a rational approach to novel therapeutic strategies.

REFERENCES

1. Gil-Sanchez A, Demmelmair H, Parrilla JJ, et al. Mechanisms involved in the selective transfer of long chain polyunsaturated fatty acids to the fetus. Front Genet 2011;2:57.
2. Larque E, Demmelmair H, Gil-Sanchez A, et al. Placental transfer of fatty acids and fetal implications. Am J Clin Nutr 2011;94:1908S–13S.
3. Pagan A, Prieto-Sanchez MT, Blanco-Carnero JE, et al. Materno-fetal transfer of docosahexaenoic acid is impaired by gestational diabetes mellitus. Am J Physiol Endocrinol Metab 2013;305:E826–33.
4. Haggarty P. Fatty acid supply to the human fetus. Annu Rev Nutr 2010;30:237–55.
5. Hanebutt FL, Demmelmair H, Schiessl B, et al. Long-chain polyunsaturated fatty acid (LC-PUFA) transfer across the placenta. Clin Nutr 2008;27:685–93.
6. Larque E, Krauss-Etschmann S, Campoy C, et al. Docosahexaenoic acid supply in pregnancy affects placental expression of fatty acid transport proteins. Am J Clin Nutr 2006;84:853–61.

7. Gil-Sanchez A, Larque E, Demmelmair H, et al. Maternal-fetal in vivo transfer of [13C]docosahexaenoic and other fatty acids across the human placenta 12 h after maternal oral intake. Am J Clin Nutr 2010;92:115–22.

8. Lapillonne A, Jensen CL. Reevaluation of the DHA requirement for the premature infant. Prostaglandins Leukot Essent Fatty Acids 2009;81:143–50.

9. O'Brien JS, Sampson EL. Lipid composition of the normal human brain: gray matter, white matter, and myelin. J Lipid Res 1965;6:537–44.

10. Lauritzen L, Hansen HS, Jorgensen MH, et al. The essentiality of long chain n-3 fatty acids in relation to development and function of the brain and retina. Prog Lipid Res 2001;40:1–94.

11. Martinez M. Tissue levels of polyunsaturated fatty acids during early human development. J Pediatr 1992;120:S129–38.

12. Su HM, Corso TN, Nathanielsz PW, et al. Linoleic acid kinetics and conversion to arachidonic acid in the pregnant and fetal baboon. J Lipid Res 1999;40:1304–12.

13. Carlson SE, Werkman SH, Peeples JM, et al. Arachidonic acid status correlates with first year growth in preterm infants. Proc Natl Acad Sci U S A 1993;90:1073–7.

14. Koletzko B, Braun M. Arachidonic acid and early human growth: is there a relation? Ann Nutr Metab 1991;35:128–31.

15. Leaf AA, Leighfield MJ, Costeloe KL, et al. Factors affecting long-chain polyunsaturated fatty acid composition of plasma choline phosphoglycerides in preterm infants. J Pediatr Gastroenterol Nutr 1992;14:300–8.

16. Martin CR, Dasilva DA, Cluette-Brown JE, et al. Decreased postnatal docosahexaenoic and arachidonic acid blood levels in premature infants are associated with neonatal morbidities. J Pediatr 2011;159:743–9.e2.

17. Vanek VW, Seidner DL, Allen P, et al. ASPEN position paper: clinical role for alternative intravenous fat emulsions. Nutr Clin Pract 2012;27:150–92.

18. Freedman SD, Blanco PG, Zaman MM, et al. Association of cystic fibrosis with abnormalities in fatty acid metabolism. N Engl J Med 2004;350:560–9.

19. Carnielli VP, Wattimena DJ, Luijendijk IH, et al. The very low birth weight premature infant is capable of synthesizing arachidonic and docosahexaenoic acids from linoleic and linolenic acids. Pediatr Res 1996;40:169–74.

20. Larque E, Demmelmair H, Koletzko B. Perinatal supply and metabolism of long-chain polyunsaturated fatty acids: importance for the early development of the nervous system. Ann N Y Acad Sci 2002;967:299–310.

21. Szitanyi P, Koletzko B, Mydlilova A, et al. Metabolism of 13C-labeled linoleic acid in newborn infants during the first week of life. Pediatr Res 1999;45:669–73.

22. Lapillonne A, Eleni dit Trolli S, Kermorvant-Duchemin E. Postnatal docosahexaenoic acid deficiency is an inevitable consequence of current recommendations and practice in preterm infants. Neonatology 2010;98:397–403.

23. Cruz-Hernandez C, Goeuriot S, Giuffrida F, et al. Direct quantification of fatty acids in human milk by gas chromatography. J Chromatogr A 2013;1284:174–9.

24. Valentine CJ, Morrow G, Fernandez S, et al. Docosahexaenoic acid and amino acid contents in pasteurized donor milk are low for preterm infants. J Pediatr 2010;157:906–10.

25. Rao JS, Ertley RN, DeMar JC Jr, et al. Dietary n-3 PUFA deprivation alters expression of enzymes of the arachidonic and docosahexaenoic acid cascades in rat frontal cortex. Mol Psychiatry 2007;12:151–7.

26. Fretham SJ, Carlson ES, Georgieff MK. Neuronal-specific iron deficiency dysregulates mammalian target of rapamycin signaling during hippocampal development in nonanemic genetic mouse models. J Nutr 2013;143:260–6.

27. Lonze BE, Ginty DD. Function and regulation of CREB family transcription factors in the nervous system. Neuron 2002;35:605–23.
28. Malamitsi-Puchner A, Economou E, Rigopoulou O, et al. Perinatal changes of brain-derived neurotrophic factor in pre- and fullterm neonates. Early Hum Dev 2004;76:17–22.
29. Sarkadi-Nagy E, Wijendran V, Diau GY, et al. The influence of prematurity and long chain polyunsaturate supplementation in 4-week adjusted age baboon neonate brain and related tissues. Pediatr Res 2003;54:244–52.
30. Manley BJ, Makrides M, Collins CT, et al. High-dose docosahexaenoic acid supplementation of preterm infants: respiratory and allergy outcomes. Pediatrics 2011;128:e71–7.
31. Skouroliakou M, Konstantinou D, Agakidis C, et al. Cholestasis, bronchopulmonary dysplasia, and lipid profile in preterm infants receiving MCT/omega-3-PUFA-containing or soybean-based lipid emulsions. Nutr Clin Pract 2012;27:817–24.
32. Ma L, Li N, Liu X, et al. Arginyl-glutamine dipeptide or docosahexaenoic acid attenuate hyperoxia-induced lung injury in neonatal mice. Nutrition 2012;28: 1186–91.
33. Rogers LK, Valentine CJ, Pennell M, et al. Maternal docosahexaenoic acid supplementation decreases lung inflammation in hyperoxia-exposed newborn mice. J Nutr 2011;141:214–22.
34. Lu J, Jilling T, Li D, et al. Polyunsaturated fatty acid supplementation alters proinflammatory gene expression and reduces the incidence of necrotizing enterocolitis in a neonatal rat model. Pediatr Res 2007;61:427–32.
35. Marion-Letellier R, Dechelotte P, Iacucci M, et al. Dietary modulation of peroxisome proliferator-activated receptor gamma. Gut 2009;58:586–93.
36. Marion-Letellier R, Savoye G, Beck PL, et al. Polyunsaturated fatty acids in inflammatory bowel diseases: a reappraisal of effects and therapeutic approaches. Inflamm Bowel Dis 2013;19:650–61.
37. Pawlik D, Lauterbach R, Walczak M, et al. Fish-oil fat emulsion supplementation reduces the risk of retinopathy in very low birth weight infants: a prospective, randomized study. JPEN J Parenter Enteral Nutr 2013. [Epub ahead of print].
38. Connor KM, SanGiovanni JP, Lofqvist C, et al. Increased dietary intake of omega-3-polyunsaturated fatty acids reduces pathological retinal angiogenesis. Nat Med 2007;13:868–73.
39. Schulzke SM, Patole SK, Simmer K. Longchain polyunsaturated fatty acid supplementation in preterm infants. Cochrane Database Syst Rev 2011;(2):CD000375.
40. Stoll BJ, Hansen NI, Adams-Chapman I, et al. Neurodevelopmental and growth impairment among extremely low-birth-weight infants with neonatal infection. JAMA 2004;292:2357–65.
41. Antonietta Ajmone-Cat M, Lavinia Salvatori M, De Simone R, et al. Docosahexaenoic acid modulates inflammatory and antineurogenic functions of activated microglial cells. J Neurosci Res 2012;90:575–87.
42. Williams JJ, Mayurasakorn K, Vannucci SJ, et al. N-3 fatty acid rich triglyceride emulsions are neuroprotective after cerebral hypoxic-ischemic injury in neonatal mice. PLoS One 2013;8:e56233.
43. D'Ascenzo R, D'Egidio S, Angelini L, et al. Parenteral nutrition of preterm infants with a lipid emulsion containing 10% fish oil: effect on plasma lipids and long-chain polyunsaturated fatty acids. J Pediatr 2011;159:33–8.e1.
44. Klein CJ, Havranek TG, Revenis ME, et al. Plasma fatty acids in premature infants with hyperbilirubinemia: before-and-after nutrition support with fish oil emulsion. Nutr Clin Pract 2013;28:87–94.

45. Torrejon C, Jung UJ, Deckelbaum RJ. n-3 Fatty acids and cardiovascular disease: actions and molecular mechanisms. Prostaglandins Leukot Essent Fatty Acids 2007;77:319–26.
46. Lapillonne A, Groh-Wargo S, Gonzalez CH, et al. Lipid needs of preterm infants: updated recommendations. J Pediatr 2013;162:S37–47.
47. Howles PN, Stemmerman GN, Fenoglio-Preiser CM, et al. Carboxyl ester lipase activity in milk prevents fat-derived intestinal injury in neonatal mice. Am J Physiol 1999;277:G653–61.
48. Makrides M. DHA supplementation during the perinatal period and neurodevelopment: do some babies benefit more than others? Prostaglandins Leukot Essent Fatty Acids 2013;88:87–90.

High-Protein Formulas
Evidence for Use in Preterm Infants

Laura D. Brown, MD[a],*, Kendra Hendrickson, MS, RD, CNSC, CSP[b], Marc L. Masor, PhD[c], William W. Hay Jr, MD[a]

KEYWORDS

- Preterm • Prematurity • Enteral feeding • Formulas • Preterm formulas
- Premature infant formulas • High-protein formulas • Protein

KEY POINTS

- Growth rates and body composition of very low birth weight preterm infants (<30 weeks' gestation, <1500 g birth weight) require 3.5 to 4.5 g/kg/d of protein in enteral formulas (or milks, mother's own or donor) at usual feeding rates (150 mL/kg/d); but the requirement for protein decreases as gestational age and birth weight advance towards term and growth rates decrease.
- Both energy and protein are required in formulas to promote growth and development, though recent studies indicate that if the protein/energy ratio in formula is too low it can promote excess fat deposition in adipose tissue that may lead to later-life obesity and associated complications.
- Deficiencies in brain, heart, lungs, liver, pancreas, kidney, and skeletal muscle have been found following preterm birth and the usual undernutrition that preterm infants receive; such deficiencies can last for the lifetime of the affected infant.
- Tables included in this article document formulas that are enriched in protein for preterm infants.

NUTRITIONAL GOALS FOR PRETERM INFANTS AND THE NEED FOR NUTRIENT-ENRICHED FORMULAS

The generally accepted goal for nutrition of the preterm infant is to achieve and maintain the growth rate and body composition of the normally growing, healthy human fetus of the same gestational age.[1] Recent efforts to meet this goal include the administration of intravenous nutrition earlier after birth and at higher rates than previously used and supplements to breast milk (mothers' own milk and donor milk); these efforts

[a] Section of Neonatology, Department of Pediatrics, Anschutz Medical Campus, University of Colorado School of Medicine, Mail Stop F441, 13243 East 23rd Avenue, Aurora, CO 80045, USA; [b] Department of Food & Nutrition, Anschutz Medical Campus, University of Colorado Hospital, Mail Stop F763, 12605 East 16th Avenue, Aurora, CO 80045, USA; [c] Clinical Nutrition Research, Abbott Nutrition, 10 Pine Ridge Loop, Durango, CO 81301, USA
* Corresponding author.
E-mail address: Laura.Brown@ucdenver.edu

Clin Perinatol 41 (2014) 383–403
http://dx.doi.org/10.1016/j.clp.2014.02.002
0095-5108/14/$ – see front matter © 2014 Elsevier Inc. All rights reserved.

are discussed elsewhere in this edition of *Clinics in Perinatology* by Stephens and Vohr in their article about protein intake and neurodevelopmental outcomes, as well as Adamkin and Radmacher in their article about the fortification of human milk for very low birth weight infants. Human milk supplemented with bovine milk–derived or human milk–derived fortifiers is the preferred enteral feeding of choice for preterm infants because of its protective effects against infection and necrotizing enterocolitis.[2–4] A mainstay of nutrition for preterm infants over the past 30 to 40 years, however, has been the use of preterm formulas or formulas designed to meet the additional protein, energy, and micronutrient requirements of the preterm infant. Preterm formulas contain more protein (2.4 g/100 mL or 3 g/100 kcal), energy (67.6–101.0 kcal/100 mL), calcium (133–146 mg/100 mL or 165–180 mg/100 kcal), and phosphorus (67–81 mg/100 mL or 83–100 mg/100 kcal) than standard formulas for term infants. New generations of high-protein preterm formulas are now available that contain even higher protein contents (2.68–2.9 g/100 mL or 3.3–3.6 g/100 kcal). Essentially all studies have documented that inadequate nutrient intakes in preterm infants have resulted in widespread postnatal growth restriction.[5,6] As a result of inadequate postnatal nutrition, infants are at risk for long-term growth and neurodevelopmental impairment.[7–11] Adequate protein intake, similar to what the fetus would receive in utero, is essential for the preterm infant to maintain growth, body composition, and nitrogen balance.

COMPLICATIONS OF INSUFFICIENT PROTEIN DELIVERY TO PRETERM INFANTS

The use of fortified human milk and/or preterm formula has resulted in greater success at achieving increased growth in weight, length, and head circumference at hospital discharge and close-to-term gestational age.[12] Such improved growth also has translated into improved, longer-term neurodevelopmental outcomes.[13–15] Nevertheless, preterm infants develop body compositions by term-corrected gestational age that are characterized by lower lean mass (LM) and relatively increased adiposity (particularly in intra-abdominal regions) in comparison with normally growing human fetuses.[16,17] Furthermore, very low birth weight (VLBW, defined as birth weight <1500 g) preterm infants experience marked linear growth suppression (stunting) that continues at least 2 years beyond hospital discharge and contributes to shorter stature even into adolescence and early adulthood.[18] A principal reason for such continued growth delays is that nutrition remains inadequate, especially in the first 2 to 4 weeks of life when physiologic instability precludes consistent protein and energy delivery.[19,20] Even when aggressive nutritional approaches are used, deficits in protein and energy still accumulate during the hospital stay of a preterm infant.[21] In addition, providing an optimal ratio of protein/energy (P/E) that fuels normal body composition is critical. If energy content of the formula is in excess relative to protein, whole-body growth can favor fat deposition over LM. On the other hand, if protein is in excess relative to energy, the excess protein may be catabolized for energy rather than to support LM growth.

Weight, length, and occipitofrontal head circumference measurements are the mainstays of monitoring growth in the neonatal intensive care unit (NICU). They are used to represent the growth and development of essentially all of the body organs in preterm infants, including the brain.[22] These measurements are positively associated with neurodevelopmental outcomes in preterm infants.[8,17,23] Conversely, poor linear growth has been implicated in worse neurodevelopmental outcomes.[11] Indeed, several studies have shown that improved nutrition with higher amounts of protein and energy intake in the postnatal period in the preterm infant correlates with increased length and head circumference at term-corrected gestational age[24–26] and with improved neurodevelopmental outcomes at 18 months corrected age.[27] For example, when more specific analysis of brain growth was measured, VLBW infants who were fed with preterm formula (increased in both energy and protein) versus regular-term infant formulas had greater caudate growth and verbal IQ at adolescence.[28,29] In another study, when preterm infants aged less than 32 weeks with evidence of white matter disease were randomized to receive 100% versus 120% of recommended average intake of protein and energy, the higher energy group had greater z scores for weight, length, head circumference, and corticospinal axonal diameter at 6 and 12 months corrected age.[30] Thus, the sequential monitoring of weight, length, and head circumference is a reasonable marker of adequate protein delivery and predictor of neurodevelopmental outcome.

Simple measurements of weight, length, and head circumference, however, likely underrepresent the specific growth deficits in lean body mass, organs, and tissues that occur as a result of suboptimal protein intake. The brain is highly reliant on protein for neuronal growth and differentiation.[31] Fetal undernutrition in animal models has been shown to restrict the growth and development of nearly every organ system in the body, including the lungs,[32] heart,[33] kidney,[34] liver,[35] pancreas,[36,37] and skeletal muscle.[38] The growth of LM depends highly on sufficient protein availability. In addition to forming the building blocks of protein within tissues, amino acids have important effects on the regulation of muscle protein synthesis and growth factor secretion. Amino acids increase skeletal muscle protein synthesis in adults, both under normal postprandial conditions as well as during catabolic states, such as after trauma or sepsis.[39,40] Increasing amino acid delivery has been shown to positively affect the net protein balance in infants born preterm or at term.[41–43] These clinical data have been corroborated by an extensive series of studies in the neonatal piglet, which have shown that both a mixed complement of amino acids and/or leucine supplementation increases muscle protein synthesis independent of other growth factor influences.[44–47] Although linear growth is a better marker for lean body mass and organ growth than weight alone,[11,48] there is still considerable need for more precise measurements of body composition, brain growth, organ size, and organ function, so that more optimal protein requirements can be met in the preterm infant population.

HOW MUCH PROTEIN IS NEEDED TO ACHIEVE NORMAL IN UTERO GROWTH RATES?

Preterm infants require greater amounts of protein to produce gestational age–appropriate rates of protein accretion than what human milk and term formulas provide.[49] Studies in normally growing fetal sheep define fractional protein synthetic and growth rates that, when scaled to human fetal growth rates, define a requirement for protein intake of 3.6 to 4.4 g/kg/d at gestational ages that would be equivalent to 24 to 30 weeks' gestational age in human fetuses.[50,51] This range encompasses the mean value of 4.0 g/kg/d of protein that is necessary to support normal human fetal growth rates at 24 to 30 weeks of gestation that was estimated by the factorial method. The factorial method uses the chemical composition of human fetuses to determine the protein and energy requirements needed to achieve fetal weight gain.[52,53] For example, protein accretion rates in the normal human fetus 24 to 30 weeks' gestation are estimated to be 1.7 g/kg/d, with lower rates as gestation progresses toward term.[54] Energy expenditure, the energy cost of growth, and the need for conversion of dietary protein into body protein increase this protein requirement to 2.5 mg/kg/d. Obligatory protein losses through the urine and skin are estimated at 0.7 to 1.0 g/kg/d. Thus, the total required enteral protein intake of a VLBW preterm infant of 24 to 30 weeks' gestation needs to be at least 3.5 to 4.0 g/kg/d (**Table 1**).[55]

Table 1
Enteral protein and energy requirements for preterm infants by the factorial approach

Body Weight (g)	Protein (g/kg/d)	Energy (kcal/kg/d)	Protein: Energy (g/100 kcal)
500–700	4.0	105	3.8
700–900	4.0	109	3.7
900–1200	4.0	119	3.4
1200–1500	3.9	127	3.1
1500–1800	3.6	128	2.8
1800–2200	3.4	131	2.6

Data from Ziegler EE. Meeting the nutritional needs of the low-birth-weight infant. Ann Nutr Metab 2011;58(Suppl 1):8–18.

Protein supply in preterm formulas must also compensate for any accumulated protein deficit, which has been observed in almost all VLBW preterm infants.[19,21,24] Some excess of protein intake over the requirements has not been shown to cause detrimental effects in preterm infants (up to 4.5 mg/kg/d, see later section). Additionally, there is consistent evidence that even a small deficit in protein will impair growth. Thus, increased formula protein concentrations are necessary to achieve a minimal overestimate of protein requirements.

Enteral protein requirements of 3.5 to 4.5 mg/kg/d for preterm infants less than 30 weeks' gestation are supported by several clinical studies that varied the amount of protein and energy and compared them with rates of neonatal growth. Ziegler[56] analyzed data from several studies published before 1986 and showed that daily weight gain increased with increasing protein delivery up to 3.6 g/kg/d. A follow-up analysis showed that protein intake ranging from 3.7 to 4.3 g/kg/d in preterm infants weighing an average of 1200 g resulted in weight gain that matches growth rates of a fetus of comparable weight (~20 g/kg/d).[57] Studies by Kashyap and colleagues[58,59] were among the first to explore the relationship between protein and energy delivery to the VLBW preterm infant by measuring daily weight gain and nitrogen retention in response to 3 different formulas with varying protein delivery (2.25–3.9 g/kg/d) and energy content (115–147 kcal/kg/d). Increased protein intake positively impacted overall body weight, length, and head circumference growth but not subcutaneous tissue estimated by triceps skinfold thickness (**Fig. 1**). At higher protein intakes, however, excess energy intake only contributed to the increased growth of body weight, largely accounted for by increased fat deposition. This landmark study can be credited for guiding the P/E ratio of standard preterm formulas (2.4 g/100 mL or 3 g/100 kcal). At a typical energy intake of 120 kcal/kg/d, standard preterm formula will provide 3.6 g/kg/d of protein.

There is still a paucity of randomized controlled clinical trials that have studied growth, nitrogen balance, body composition, and long-term neurodevelopmental outcomes related to different protein intakes in preterm infants. A Cochrane review in 2006 compiled the randomized controlled trials available that contrasted levels of formula protein intakes defined as low (<3.0 g/kg/d), high (between 3.0 and 4.0 g/kg/d), and very high (>4.0 g/kg/d) in neonates with a birth weight less than 2500 g. This review included 5 randomized controlled trials (including the studies of Kashyap and colleagues[58,59] previously mentioned) and concluded that when protein intakes are high while other nutrients are kept constant, weight gain and nitrogen accretion are improved.[26] Because of the limited available evidence, however, specific recommendations could not be made for the administration of very-high-protein intakes

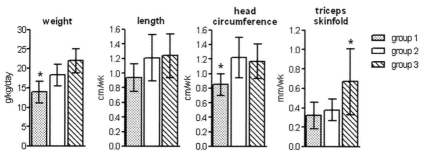

Fig. 1. Growth rates with varying protein and energy intakes. Weight, length, head circumference, and triceps skinfold thickness were determined serially in preterm infants with a birthweight of 900 to 1750 g fed one of 3 formulas which provided the following protein and energy intakes: 2.24 g/kg/d and 115 kcal/kg/d (group 1, *dotted bars*), 3.6 g/kg/d and 115 kcal/kg/d (group 2, *clear bars*), and 3.5 g/kg/d and 149 kcal/kg/d (group 3, *striped bars*). Weight gain and rate of increase in length and head circumference were less in group 1 than in groups 2 and 3. The rate of weight gain was not significantly greater in group 3 than in group 2, but the rate of increase in skinfold thickness was greater in group 3. * Significantly different from other 2 groups (P<0.05). (*Adapted from* Kashyap S, Forsyth M, Zucker C, et al. Effects of varying protein and energy intakes on growth and metabolic response in low birth weight infants. J Pediatr 1986;108(6):958; with permission.)

(>4.0 g/kg/d) and conclusions could not be made about the effects of protein delivery on the long-term neurodevelopmental outcome. A representative study by Fairey and colleagues,[60] who randomized preterm infants to receive preterm infant formula with 3.2 versus 2.6 g of protein/100 kcal, found no difference in net nitrogen retention or partitioning of stored energy as protein and fat. Perhaps neither of these formulas provided sufficient protein for growth relative to energy, diminishing the impact of the so-called greater protein intake used in these studies. Essentially all other studies have shown improved growth with higher protein intake in the formulas used. For example, Cooke and colleagues[61] randomized preterm infants with birth weights less than 1500 g to receive preterm infant formula with higher protein content (3.0 vs 3.6 g of protein/100 kcal) in a balanced crossover design study. Increased protein accretion and improved weight gain without evidence of metabolic stress were observed when infants received a protein content of 3.6 g/100 kcal. These conclusions are further supported by several studies that, either retrospectively or prospectively, compared improved or aggressive nutritional practice changes to historical approaches. These studies included minimum rates of protein delivery of 3.5 g/kg/d. Consistently, improved weight, length, and head circumference measurements were observed with increased energy and protein delivery,[25,62,63] with specific improvements in LM.[64]

It is important to recognize that at more advanced gestational ages, normal fetal fractional protein synthetic rates and growth rates decline, reducing the requirement for protein intake. At approximately 36 weeks' gestation, growth rates decline toward those of the normal full-term infant, whose protein requirements are in the range of 1.5 to 2.0 g/kg/d seen in data from fetal sheep (**Fig. 2**).[65] The potential benefit of increased protein and energy intake from preterm formulas may become less significant at more mature gestational ages, provided that the total intake of milk or 20-kcal term infant formulas that contain approximately 2% protein reaches or exceeds 150 mL/kg/d and, thus, provides sufficient protein intake.[66] For the late preterm infant born at 34 weeks' gestation or greater, standard term formula (if human milk is not available) ingested in

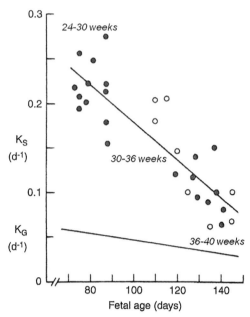

Fig. 2. Fractional rate of protein synthesis (K_S) over the course of gestation in fetal sheep. Fetal sheep at varying gestational ages (term 145 days) were infused with leucine (*filled circle*) and lysine (*open circle*) radioactive tracers to determine K_S (grams of protein per kilogram of body weight per day) and compared with the fractional rate of growth (K_G) (grams of body weight per kilograms per day). Equivalent time periods during human gestation are shown in italics. These data show that both the fractional rates of protein synthesis and growth decrease between 30 and 36 weeks' gestation, as does the protein requirement for growth. (*From* Hay WW Jr, Regnault TR, Brown LD. Fetal requirements and placental transfer of nitrogenous compounds. In: Polin RA, Fox WW, Abman SH, editors. Fetal and neonatal physiology. 4th edition. Philadelphia: Saunders, an imprint of Elsevier, Inc; 2011. p. 595; with permission.)

adequate volumes might be sufficient. However, a significant amount of brain development occurs between 34 and 40 weeks' gestation, including a 50% increase in cortical volume,[67] which could be compromised if suboptimal amounts of protein are delivered. Furthermore, brain growth in the late preterm infant is particularly vulnerable if growth is compromised by illness. Therefore, more than 2 g/kg/d of protein might be required to achieve appropriate gestational age–specific fractional protein synthesis and growth rates in the late preterm infant. For infants born between 24 and 30 weeks' gestation, nutrient-enriched transitional formulas are recommended after discharge through 6 to 9 months corrected age because most of these infants have considerable protein and energy deficits even at term-corrected gestational age.[68,69] Use of a transitional formula for 6 months after discharge versus standard term formula in VLBW infants has been shown to increase LM without increasing percent body fat at 1 year[70] and decrease body fat, truncal fat, and fasting insulin concentrations at 2 years.[71]

NEED FOR ADDITIONAL ENERGY AS WELL AS PROTEIN IN HIGH-PROTEIN FORMULAS

Nearly all formulas with higher concentrations of protein also have increased caloric density from additional carbohydrate and lipid. Both energy and protein intakes are beneficial for growth of body weight, length, and head circumference. Energy intake is required for the synthesis and deposition protein and fat or, in other words, the energy cost of growth.[72] Preterm infants need a minimum of 110 kcal/kg/d to maintain the growth of adipose tissue that is observed in the normally growing human fetus.[73] A series of controlled enteral feeding studies in preterm infants further examined the effects of relative protein and energy intake on the rate and composition of weight gain.[58,59] In general, relatively more protein was synthesized and deposited in growing lean tissue at higher protein intakes and more fat was synthesized and deposited in growth of adipose tissue at higher energy intakes. Slightly higher amounts of energy, more than 100 kcal/kg/d, were needed to promote lean body growth at the in utero rate. Thus, a caloric intake of 115 to 120 kcal/kg/d will appropriately support a protein intake of 3.5 to 4.0 g/kg/d; more energy produces more body fat gain, but more protein than 4 g/kg/d does not independently increase LM gain (**Fig. 3**),[74] supporting that excess protein relative to energy is catabolized rather than used for LM growth.

Thus, there is no apparent benefit of an energy intake in excess of that necessary to assure utilization of the concomitant protein intake. Excessive energy and carbohydrate intakes simply result in excessive fat deposition relative to protein deposition. In fact, evidence indicates that changes in body composition in preterm infants during their NICU days demonstrate a relatively greater gain in body fat than would have occurred had these infants remained in utero.[16,53,75] The potential for such rapid gains in adiposity may lead to later-life obesity and associated complications.[48,76] These observations account for recent efforts to enhance the P/E ratio of the diets of preterm infants, particularly to add more protein supplements to maternal and especially mature donor breast milk.[77]

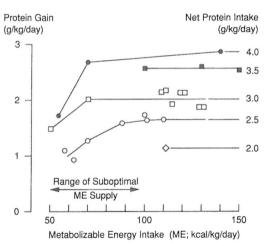

Fig. 3. Protein needs of the preterm infant. In a group of VLBW preterm infants, the effect of increasing energy intake on protein gain at different protein intakes (2.0 [*diamond*], 2.5 [*open circle*], 3.0 [*open square*], 3.5 [*filled square*], and 4.0 [*filled circle*] g/kg/d) was determined. In the range of suboptimal energy intake (50–90 kcal/kg/d) and lower protein intake (2.5 g/kg/d), protein gain can be improved by increasing energy intakes. At 3.0 and 4.0 g of protein per kilogram per day, energy increases beyond 70 kcal/kg/d added no more body protein. With energy intakes more than 100 kcal/kg/d, there was minimal further positive effect on protein gain regardless of protein intake. (*From* Micheli JL, Schutz Y. Protein. In: Tsang RC, Lucas A, Uauy R, et al, editors. Nutritional needs of the preterm infant. 1st edition. Pawling (NY): Caduceus Medical Publishers; 1993. p. 35.)

POTENTIAL COMPLICATIONS OF HIGH-PROTEIN DELIVERY

To meet the greater needs for protein and energy required for promoting growth and development, preterm formulas, enriched relative to human milk and term infant formulas, have been developed and have become a mainstay of nutrition of preterm infants. Development and widespread use of such formulas began more than 40 years ago. Even the first protein-enriched formulas were quite successful at promoting nitrogen balance and growth. However, there was significant concern for adverse outcomes of high-protein administration to preterm infants.[78–80] The classic studies in this regard by Goldman and colleagues[81–83] added bovine casein to produce 4% versus standard 2% protein concentrations in the formulas, providing up to 6.0 to 7.2 g/kg/d of protein in the supplemented group versus 3.0 to 3.6 g/kg/d in the standard formulas. Most of the infants enrolled in these studies were born between 1500 and 2000 g, which is in a weight and corresponding gestational age range that would not require such high rates of protein intake. Furthermore, a large proportion (~50%) of the population was born small for gestational age (SGA, <10% of weight for gestational age). If these SGA infants were small because of intrauterine growth restriction (IUGR), it is quite likely that higher protein intakes would not have been well tolerated because of slower growth potential. Not surprisingly, therefore, several adverse outcomes were associated with the higher protein intake of the supplemented group, including metabolic acidosis, fever, poor growth, higher-than-normal plasma amino acid concentrations, and later developmental delays. Such adverse outcomes primarily occurred among those infants enrolled in the studies who had birth weights less than 1300 g. Not only was the 6- to 7-g/kg/d protein supply far greater than needed by the healthy growing human fetus of earlier gestational age but also much in excess of the protein requirements for older preterm infants more than 30 weeks' gestation. Indeed, Kashyap and colleagues[58] produced in utero growth in preterm infants of this same gestational age and slightly younger with 3.5 g/kg/d of protein in the enteral diet.

More recent evidence of protein overload has been reported in preterm infants fed a formula with a P/E ratio of 3.6 g/100 kcal that provided absolute protein intakes of 4.3 g/kg/d and energy intakes of 120 kcal/kg/d.[58] This study reported higher blood urea nitrogen (BUN) concentrations (mean 10.5 mg/dL) as well as plasma threonine and tyrosine concentrations of more than 2 SD more than the mean umbilical cord plasma concentrations of infants born at similar gestational ages. However, in a more recent study, VLBW preterm infants fed a formula with the same P/E ratio and receiving absolute mean protein intakes of 4.6 g/kg/d for 1 week had no evidence of metabolic stress.[61] The investigators of this study acknowledged that the duration of the intervention was short, and it is unknown whether longer-term feeding of a high P/E ratio might affect the metabolic status of these infants. Therefore, the upper limit of protein intake and the ideal P/E ratio remain controversial. Current evidence supports the beneficial and safe use of formulas providing a P/E ratio of 3.2 to 3.3 g/100 kcal. At an energy intake of 120 kcal/kg/d, a preterm formula with a P/E ratio of 3.2 to 3.3 g/100 kcal provides protein intake of 3.8 to 4.0 g/kg/d.[56,57,84] There is still a great need, however, for longitudinal studies to assess the effects of these intakes on long-term outcomes of growth, body composition, neurodevelopment, and clinical susceptibility to adult-onset diseases.

Concerns for metabolic acidosis from high-protein delivery persist, though not from studies or experience using preterm, higher-protein formulas but from supplementing human milk with a new, higher-protein bovine liquid human milk fortifier that was acidified to provide commercial sterility (successful aseptic processing in extremely small volumes had not been achieved at the time this fortifier was introduced). One randomized, third party–masked, multicentered published study demonstrated improved growth and no differences for other potential complications among infants fed the liquid protein supplement versus those fed a standard powdered human milk supplement.[77] There were, however, indications of more acidity, including significantly lower pH at 6 days, lower bicarbonate at 6 and 14 days, lower carbon dioxide (CO_2) at 14 and 28 days, and higher chloride at 14 and 28 days. Although in the normal range, all of these changes were in the direction of a more acidic physiology. Two additional studies (one randomized and only documented in abstract form and the other retrospective) showed slower rates of growth and lower serum CO_2 concentrations and greater base deficits as evidence of increased metabolic acidosis among infants fed the acidified liquid fortifier compared with other infants fed powdered human milk fortifier.[85,86] The evidence, therefore, remains insufficient to determine whether an extra acid load used for the purpose of sterility could be detrimental or not.

High concentrations of a single amino acid or a select few amino acids can interfere with the uptake of amino acids by the brain and other organs and protein synthesis. Despite the importance of achieving an appropriate balance of the serum amino acid profile, only a few studies of infants receiving preterm formulas with protein delivery of 3.5 to 4.0 g/kg/d have measured plasma amino acid concentrations. Studies that are available show that for most amino acids, their concentrations are similar to what would be found in umbilical cord blood, with the exception of slightly higher threonine and tyrosine concentrations.[59,87] It is more likely that the quality of protein influences the balance of amino acid concentrations because the whey-to-casein ratio affects individual amino acid intakes. When preterm infants received study formulas that varied the ratio of whey to casein, the plasma concentrations of several amino acid concentrations differed, though no difference was observed in acid-base status.[88] Notably, plasma threonine concentrations were increased and phenylalanine and tyrosine concentrations were decreased in infants fed whey-predominant formula compared with those fed casein-predominant formula.[58,88] This effect would be exacerbated in 100%-whey preterm formulas, which are partially hydrolyzed (such as Gerber Good Start Premature 24, Nestlé, Vevey, Switzerland (see **Table 3**)). Large neutral amino acids (LNAA) such as tyrosine and phenylalanine are precursors for neurotransmitters and compete for the LNAA transporter across the blood-brain barrier. Plasma amino acid profiles also vary between preterm infants receiving fortified human milk versus preterm formula, which contain different whey-to-casien ratios.[89] In contrast, attention has shifted to studies of intravenous feeding whereby almost universally total amino acid infusion rates of 3 to 4 g/kg/d have shown plasma amino acid concentrations less than or equal to umbilical venous plasma amino acid concentrations in normally growing human fetuses of the same gestational age.[43,90–92] Such intravenous nutrition studies have also shown modest and appropriate increases in BUN, no significant increases in ammonia concentrations, and no significant metabolic acidosis.[93]

PROTEIN AND ENERGY REQUIREMENTS FOR THE INFANT BORN WITH IUGR

Protein and energy requirements for the infant born with IUGR from insufficient placental nutrient supply require special consideration. These infants are often born both preterm and SGA. Placental insufficiency produces chronic fetal growth restriction, as evidenced by abnormal Doppler flow studies with high resistive indices in the umbilical vessels, shunting of blood flow to vital organs, and preserved head circumference.[94,95] Selective redistribution of blood flow away from musculoskeletal structures results in decreased LM and fat mass at the time of birth.[96,97] Because of the lack of published data about the nutritional requirements of this population, recommendations for the nutritional management of the SGA infant are not distinguished from appropriate for gestational age (AGA) preterm infants.[98]

However, IUGR neonates born preterm represent a true nutritional challenge. The goal is still to provide sufficient nutrients to achieve postnatal growth similar to that of a normal fetus of matched gestational age, especially because they are at higher risk of poorer neurodevelopmental outcome than AGA preterm infants.[99] However, rapid catch-up growth, especially by providing additional energy without parallel increases in linear and LM growth, might increase the longer-term risk for metabolic complications, including visceral obesity, insulin resistance, and type 2 diabetes.[100] Little is known about how an IUGR neonate handles higher protein supplementation. A study in 1988 by Boehm and colleagues[101] showed that with protein intakes of more than 2.5 g/kg/d, SGA infants had higher alpha-amino-nitrogen in the serum and urine as well as total bile acid concentrations in the serum when compared with AGA infants. The differences between SGA and AGA infants became more pronounced with an increasing protein intake, suggesting that SGA infants are more sensitive to an excessive protein intake than AGA infants. Another trial randomized term SGA neonates to a nutrient-enriched versus standard formula and found a slightly lower psychomotor developmental index at 9 months of age in those infants receiving the enriched formula.[102] It is possible that postnatal hepatic clearance of amino acids might be compromised because of chronic reductions in hepatic blood flow in utero from reduced umbilical blood flow and dilation of the ductus venosus that would shunt umbilical blood flow past the liver.[103] Future research is needed to determine optimal protein and energy requirements in this unique population of infants.

QUALITY OF PROTEIN IN PRETERM FORMULAS

The ratio of whey to casein protein in formulas affects protein absorption, metabolism, and concentrations of circulating amino acids. Thus, it is an important consideration when defining protein requirements for the preterm infant. Bovine milk protein is casein predominant (whey-to-casein ratio of 18:82), whereas human milk protein is whey predominant (whey-to-casein ratio of 70:30), although the actual whey-to-casein ratio of human milk is quite variable.[104] Most formulas have been modified to more closely match the protein composition of human milk and, therefore, have whey-to-casein ratios of 60:40. Indeed, when optimization studies were done with cow milk protein, a whey-to-casein ratio of 48:52 was found to produce plasma amino acid concentrations in formula-fed term infants that most closely approximated those of the term breast-fed infant.[105] However, the absolute concentrations of amino acids in the more rapidly growing fetus are higher than slower-growing, breast-fed term infants. For preterm formulas, a higher amount of protein as well as a greater whey-to-casein ratio are needed to achieve both growth and appropriate plasma amino acid concentrations.

Preterm infants fed formula with a whey-to-casein protein ratio of 60:40 have well-balanced plasma amino acids and adequate protein utilization.[87] Higher proportions of casein cannot be handled with the same efficiency, as shown by the development of metabolic acidosis and higher plasma tyrosine and phenylalanine concentrations reported with formulas derived from bovine milk with a 18:82 whey-to-casein ratio.[106–109] The complement of amino acids derived from protein digestion and absorption are important, not just for provision of sufficient amounts of essential amino acids but also because the balance among individual amino acids seems to be important for producing normal cellular development and function, particularly in the brain. As discussed earlier, the type of protein used in preterm formulas may change the levels of specific amino acids.[88] The whey fraction provides lower concentrations of phenylalanine, tyrosine, and methionine and higher concentrations of taurine compared with the casein fraction; these amino acid patterns are reflected in blood concentrations. Taurine in cow's milk is low, which is why both term and preterm formulas are supplemented with taurine.[110] Unfortunately, there still is a paucity of information about optimal intakes of specific amino acids for the preterm infant.

Earlier casein-predominant formulas also produced complications of feeding intolerance and, in some cases, lactobezoars in LBW infants.[111] These complications might have been because casein more easily coagulates when acidified in the stomach. However, as a result of partial coagulation, casein digestion is slower than with whey protein. Casein protein produces a slower increase in plasma amino acid concentrations over a longer period of time because of slower gastric emptying and digestion.[112] Whey protein produces a more rapid increase in plasma amino acid concentrations but for a shorter duration. Differences in absorption rates based on the whey-to-casein ratio could have important effects on amino acid metabolism. In adults, a more rapid increase in amino acids from the digestion of whey protein will preferentially increase protein synthesis and amino acid oxidation, whereas slow and sustained absorption of casein protein will have a greater effect on the reduction of protein breakdown.[112]

Such studies have not been conducted in preterm infants. However, animal studies indicate that there may be similar responses to the duration of gastric emptying and digestion in such infants, with greater protein synthesis produced by feedings that produced rapid increases in plasma amino acid concentrations. For example, in neonatal piglets, Davis and colleagues showed that intermittent bolus feedings enhanced muscle protein synthesis greater than continuous feedings,[113,114] as did leucine boluses during continuous feedings.[115] In the clinical setting, feeding tolerance is generally increased by intermittent, bolus feedings versus continuous feedings in preterm infants.[116] These studies lend support to the benefit of using more rapidly digestible whey protein formulas to promote protein synthesis and lean body mass growth in the preterm infant.

In this regard, preterm formulas are available with 100% whey partially hydrolyzed protein and are marketed to improve enteral feeding tolerance by enhancing amino acid absorption into the circulation. However, such potential benefits of improved amino acid absorption are controversial, as there is evidence that hydrolyzed protein is not used as efficiently as intact protein.[117,118] Instead, hydrolyzed protein in human milk fortifiers and the use of relatively hydrolyzed protein in selected infant formulas (the Gerber preterm formula line and non–preterm formulas, such as Pregestimil from Mead Johnson Nutrition [Evansville, IN] and Alimentum from Abbott Nutrition [Abbott Park, IL]) have primarily been used when gut developmental defects

Table 2
Recommended enteral macronutrient intakes for VLBW preterm infants (<1500 g)

	Protein (g/kg/d)	Energy (kcal/kg/d)	Protein/Energy (g/100 kcal)
ESPGHAN	3.5–4.5[a]	110–130	2.25–3.1
LSRO	3.4–4.3	110–135	2.5–3.6
Canadian Pediatric Society	3.0–4.0[b]	105–135	2.5–3.0
AAP Committee on Nutrition	3.5–4.0	105–130	2.9–3.3

[a] Protein intake of 4.0 to 4.5 g/kg/d for infants weighing less than 1000 g.
[b] Protein intake of 3.5 to 4.0 g/kg/d for infants weighing less than 1000 g.

Table 3
Composition of preterm formulas

	Protein (g/100 mL)	Calcium (mg/100 mL)	Phosphorus (mg/100 mL)	Zinc (mg/100 mL)	Protein/Energy (g/100 Kcal)	Protein Source
Standard Preterm Formulas						
Enfamil Premature 24 with Iron (Mead Johnson Nutrition)	2.4	134	67	1.2	3.0	60% whey 40% casein[a]
Gerber Good Start Premature 24	2.4	133	69	1.1	3.0	100% whey partially hydrolyzed[a]
Similac Special Care 24 (Abbott Nutrition)	2.4	146	81	1.2	3.0	60% whey 40% casein[a]
High-Protein Formulas						
Enfamil Premature 24 Cal High Protein	2.8	134	67	1.2	3.5	60% whey 40% casein[a]
Gerber Good Start Premature 24 High Protein	2.9	133	69	1.1	3.6	100% whey partially hydrolyzed[a]
Similac Special Care 24 High Protein	2.7	146	81	1.2	3.3	60% whey 40% casein[a]
International Formulas						
Milupa Aptamil Preterm (Wiltshire, England)	2.6	94	62	1.1	3.3	60% whey 40% casein[a]
Nestlé Partially Hydrolyzed Premature (Nestlé)	2.9	116	77	1.2	3.6	100% whey partially hydrolyzed[a]
Cow & Gate Nutriprem 1 Low Birthweight (Cuijk, the Netherlands)	2.6	94	62	1.1	3.3	61% whey 39% casein[a]

[a] From nonfat milk and whey protein concentrate.

(gastroschisis) or injuries (necrotizing enterocolitis, inflammation reactions to bovine milk antigen) have limited digestive capacities.

HOW DO YOU CHOOSE THE RIGHT PROTEIN DELIVERY FOR YOUR PATIENT?

After an extensive review of the literature, several expert panels and committees have made recommendations for protein, energy, and P/E balance that VLBW preterm infants (<1500 g) should receive from enteral feeding. Recommendations from the European Society for Pediatric Gastroenterology, Hepatology, and Nutrition (ESPGHAN) Committee on Nutrition,[119] Canadian Pediatric Society,[120] American Academy of Pediatrics Committee on Nutrition (AAP),[121] and the Expert Panel for the American Society of Nutritional Sciences Life Sciences Research Office (LSRO)[122] are listed in **Table 2**. The recommended range of protein intake from the ESPGHAN Committee on Nutrition is 3.8 to 4.5 g/kg/d for infants up to 1000 g and 3.5 to 4.0 g for infants from 1000 to 1800 g.[119] LSRO concluded that the minimum protein intake of premature infants is 3.4 g/kg/d and that a protein intake of 4.3 g/kg/d is without adverse consequences. There is a gap in the recommendations for preterm infants with a birth weight of more than 1800 g or more than 30 weeks' gestational age, with little experimental evidence to support goals for protein, energy, mineral, and micronutrient needs for the intermediate to late preterm infant. Further research is very much needed for this largest portion of the population of preterm infants to establish a rational basis for their optimal nutrition.

Several formulas available in North America are marketed as either regular protein content or high protein content (**Table 3**). International formulas contain relatively higher protein content in their standard preterm infant formulas. They do not, however, have a high-protein designation, perhaps related to the higher minimum protein intakes recommended by the 2010 guidelines from the ESPGHAN for preterm infants weighing less than 1000 g used in Europe when compared with the 2002 guidelines from the LSRO used in the United States. The source of protein is similar between all products with the exception of the Gerber formula, which is 100% whey and partially hydrolyzed. The micronutrients in the North American formulas vary by more than 10% in many cases, whereas the international formulas shown are almost identical in composition. When feeding a 120-kcal/kg/d diet, standard preterm

---

Box 1
Indications for using high-protein preterm formulas

Weight less than 1500 g

Fluid/volume-restricted infants

Promotion of wound healing

Cumulative deficit of protein intake

   Prolonged peripheral parenteral nutrition (limited protein content)

   Inadequate parenteral nutrition caused by fluid restriction

   History of feeding intolerance resulting in interruption of enteral feeds

   Multiple procedures/surgeries resulting in interruption of enteral feeds

Inadequate growth in length and/or head circumference

Partial unfortified human milk feeds (eg, direct breastfeeding)

Lower energy needs but higher protein needs

formulas provide 3.6 g/kg/d of protein, whereas high-protein formulas provide a range of 3.9 to 4.35 g/kg/d of protein. There are several clinical circumstances that may warrant the use of high-protein formulas for preterm infants in the NICU, which are listed in **Box 1**.

SUMMARY

High-protein, preterm formulas serve an important role in ensuring adequate nutrient and protein delivery to the VLBW preterm infant, especially when human milk is unavailable. Nutritional goals in the NICU are to match protein requirements for fractional rates of protein synthesis and growth of the fetus of equivalent weight and gestational age. There is sufficient evidence to support high-protein delivery in the range of 3.0 to 4.5 g/kg/d to VLBW (<1500 g) and extremely low birthweight (<1000 g) infants. The quantity of protein delivery depends on the gestational age, birthweight, and cumulative deficits in protein delivery that a preterm infant experiences. There still are gaps in knowledge regarding the quality of protein that should be fed to the preterm infant (balance of whey and casein, need for hydrolyzed protein) as studies that measure the plasma amino acid profiles in rapidly growing VLBW infants are limited. The consequences of inadequate protein delivery are significant and are directly related to long-term neurocognitive as well as metabolic outcomes. Therefore, meticulous attention to quantity and quality of protein delivery to the preterm infant has the potential to improve lean mass growth, neurodevelopment, and metabolic health in this high-risk population.

ACKNOWLEDGMENTS

The authors wish to thank Bonnie Savone for her tireless effort at article organization. This work was supported by the NIH-K12-HD057022 Building Interdisciplinary Research Careers in Women's Health (L.D. Brown), University of Colorado Center for Women's Health Research (L.D. Brown), NIH-K12-HD068372 Child Health Research Career Development Award (W.W. Hay Jr), NIH-UL1-RR025780 Colorado Clinical and Translational Science Institute (W.W. Hay Jr), NIH-T32-HD007186-32 Training in Perinatal Medicine and Biology (W.W. Hay Jr), NIH-R01-DK088139 Research Project Award (W.W. Hay Jr), and The Bill and Melinda Gates Foundation OPP1061082 Grand Challenges Explorations (W.W. Hay Jr).

REFERENCES

1. American Academy of Pediatrics Committee on Nutrition: nutritional needs of low-birth-weight infants. Pediatrics 1985;75(5):976–86.
2. Cristofalo EA, Schanler RJ, Blanco CL, et al. Randomized trial of exclusive human milk versus preterm formula diets in extremely premature infants. J Pediatr 2013;163(6):1592–5.
3. Schanler RJ, Shulman RJ, Lau C. Feeding strategies for premature infants: beneficial outcomes of feeding fortified human milk versus preterm formula. Pediatrics 1999;103(6 Pt 1):1150–7.
4. Schanler RJ. Mother's own milk, donor human milk, and preterm formulas in the feeding of extremely premature infants. J Pediatr Gastroenterol Nutr 2007; 45(Suppl 3):S175–7.
5. Clark RH, Thomas P, Peabody J. Extrauterine growth restriction remains a serious problem in prematurely born neonates. Pediatrics 2003;111(5 Pt 1): 986–90.

6. Stoll BJ, Hansen NI, Bell EF, et al. Neonatal outcomes of extremely preterm infants from the NICHD Neonatal Research Network. Pediatrics 2010;126(3): 443–56.
7. Ehrenkranz RA, Dusick AM, Vohr BR, et al. Growth in the neonatal intensive care unit influences neurodevelopmental and growth outcomes of extremely low birth weight infants. Pediatrics 2006;117(4):1253–61.
8. Franz AR, Pohlandt F, Bode H, et al. Intrauterine, early neonatal, and postdischarge growth and neurodevelopmental outcome at 5.4 years in extremely preterm infants after intensive neonatal nutritional support. Pediatrics 2009;123(1):e101–9.
9. Hack M, Breslau N, Weissman B, et al. Effect of very low birth weight and subnormal head size on cognitive abilities at school age. N Engl J Med 1991;325(4): 231–7.
10. Latal-Hajnal B, von SK, Kovari H, et al. Postnatal growth in VLBW infants: significant association with neurodevelopmental outcome. J Pediatr 2003;143(2): 163–70.
11. Ramel SE, Demerath EW, Gray HL, et al. The relationship of poor linear growth velocity with neonatal illness and two-year neurodevelopment in preterm infants. Neonatology 2012;102(1):19–24.
12. Wilson DC, Cairns P, Halliday HL, et al. Randomised controlled trial of an aggressive nutritional regimen in sick very low birthweight infants. Arch Dis Child Fetal Neonatal Ed 1997;77(1):F4–11.
13. Lucas A, Morley R, Cole TJ, et al. Early diet in preterm babies and developmental status in infancy. Arch Dis Child 1989;64(11):1570–8.
14. Lucas A, Morley R, Cole TJ. Randomised trial of early diet in preterm babies and later intelligence quotient. BMJ 1998;317(7171):1481–7.
15. Tyson JE, Lasky RE, Mize CE, et al. Growth, metabolic response, and development in very-low-birth-weight infants fed banked human milk or enriched formula. I. Neonatal findings. J Pediatr 1983;103(1):95–104.
16. Johnson MJ, Wootton SA, Leaf AA, et al. Preterm birth and body composition at term equivalent age: a systematic review and meta-analysis. Pediatrics 2012; 130(3):e640–9.
17. Ramel SE, Gray HL, Ode KL, et al. Body composition changes in preterm infants following hospital discharge: comparison with term infants. J Pediatr Gastroenterol Nutr 2011;53(3):333–8.
18. Paz I, Seidman DS, Danon YL, et al. Are children born small for gestational age at increased risk of short stature? Am J Dis Child 1993;147(3):337–9.
19. Embleton NE, Pang N, Cooke RJ. Postnatal malnutrition and growth retardation: an inevitable consequence of current recommendations in preterm infants? Pediatrics 2001;107(2):270–3.
20. Ernst KD, Radmacher PG, Rafail ST, et al. Postnatal malnutrition of extremely low birth-weight infants with catch-up growth postdischarge. J Perinatol 2003;23(6): 477–82.
21. Dinerstein A, Nieto RM, Solana CL, et al. Early and aggressive nutritional strategy (parenteral and enteral) decreases postnatal growth failure in very low birth weight infants. J Perinatol 2006;26(7):436–42.
22. Skullerud K. Variations in the size of the human brain. Influence of age, sex, body length, body mass index, alcoholism, Alzheimer changes, and cerebral atherosclerosis. Acta Neurol Scand Suppl 1985;102:1–94.
23. Belfort MB, Rifas-Shiman SL, Sullivan T, et al. Infant growth before and after term: effects on neurodevelopment in preterm infants. Pediatrics 2011;128(4): e899–906.

24. Can E, Bulbul A, Uslu S, et al. Effects of aggressive parenteral nutrition on growth and clinical outcome in preterm infants. Pediatr Int 2012;54(6):869–74.

25. Cormack BE, Bloomfield FH. Increased protein intake decreases postnatal growth faltering in ELBW babies. Arch Dis Child Fetal Neonatal Ed 2013; 98(5):F399–404.

26. Premji SS, Fenton TR, Sauve RS. Higher versus lower protein intake in formula-fed low birth weight infants. Cochrane Database Syst Rev 2006;(1):CD003959.

27. Stephens BE, Walden RV, Gargus RA, et al. First-week protein and energy intakes are associated with 18-month developmental outcomes in extremely low birth weight infants. Pediatrics 2009;123(5):1337–43.

28. Isaacs EB, Gadian DG, Sabatini S, et al. The effect of early human diet on caudate volumes and IQ. Pediatr Res 2008;63(3):308–14.

29. Isaacs EB, Morley R, Lucas A. Early diet and general cognitive outcome at adolescence in children born at or below 30 weeks gestation. J Pediatr 2009; 155(2):229–34.

30. Dabydeen L, Thomas JE, Aston TJ, et al. High-energy and -protein diet increases brain and corticospinal tract growth in term and preterm infants after perinatal brain injury. Pediatrics 2008;121(1):148–56.

31. Fuglestad AJ, Rao R, Georgieff MK. The role of nutrition in cognitive development. In: Nelson CA, Luciana L, editors. Handbook of developmental cognitive neuroscience. 2nd edition. Cambridge (United Kingdom): MIT Press; 2008. p. 623–42.

32. Rozance PJ, Seedorf GJ, Brown A, et al. Intrauterine growth restriction decreases pulmonary alveolar and vessel growth and causes pulmonary artery endothelial cell dysfunction in vitro in fetal sheep. Am J Physiol Lung Cell Mol Physiol 2011;301(6):L860–71.

33. Corstius HB, Zimanyi MA, Maka N, et al. Effect of intrauterine growth restriction on the number of cardiomyocytes in rat hearts. Pediatr Res 2005;57(6):796–800.

34. Woods LL, Ingelfinger JR, Nyengaard JR, et al. Maternal protein restriction suppresses the newborn renin-angiotensin system and programs adult hypertension in rats. Pediatr Res 2001;49(4):460–7.

35. He ZX, Wu DQ, Sun ZH, et al. Protein or energy restriction during late gestation alters fetal growth and visceral organ mass: an evidence of intrauterine programming in goats. Anim Reprod Sci 2013;137(3–4):177–82.

36. Cherif H, Reusens B, Dahri S, et al. A protein-restricted diet during pregnancy alters in vitro insulin secretion from islets of fetal Wistar rats. J Nutr 2001; 131(5):1555–9.

37. Snoeck A, Remacle C, Reusens B, et al. Effect of a low protein diet during pregnancy on the fetal rat endocrine pancreas. Biol Neonate 1990;57(2):107–18.

38. De Blasio MJ, Gatford KL, Robinson JS, et al. Placental restriction of fetal growth reduces size at birth and alters postnatal growth, feeding activity, and adiposity in the young lamb. Am J Physiol Regul Integr Comp Physiol 2007;292(2): R875–86.

39. Drummond MJ, Rasmussen BB. Leucine-enriched nutrients and the regulation of mammalian target of rapamycin signalling and human skeletal muscle protein synthesis. Curr Opin Clin Nutr Metab Care 2008;11(3):222–6.

40. Wolfe RR. Regulation of skeletal muscle protein metabolism in catabolic states. Curr Opin Clin Nutr Metab Care 2005;8(1):61–5.

41. Poindexter BB, Karn CA, Ahlrichs JA, et al. Amino acids suppress proteolysis independent of insulin throughout the neonatal period. Am J Physiol 1997; 272(4 Pt 1):E592–9.

42. Reynolds RM, Bass KD, Thureen PJ. Achieving positive protein balance in the immediate postoperative period in neonates undergoing abdominal surgery. J Pediatr 2008;152(1):63–7.
43. Thureen PJ, Melara D, Fennessey PV, et al. Effect of low versus high intravenous amino acid intake on very low birth weight infants in the early neonatal period. Pediatr Res 2003;53(1):24–32.
44. O'Connor PM, Kimball SR, Suryawan A, et al. Regulation of translation initiation by insulin and amino acids in skeletal muscle of neonatal pigs. Am J Physiol Endocrinol Metab 2003;285(1):E40–53.
45. O'Connor PM, Bush JA, Suryawan A, et al. Insulin and amino acids independently stimulate skeletal muscle protein synthesis in neonatal pigs. Am J Physiol Endocrinol Metab 2003;284(1):E110–9.
46. Suryawan A, Jeyapalan AS, Orellana RA, et al. Leucine stimulates protein synthesis in skeletal muscle of neonatal pigs by enhancing mTORC1 activation. Am J Physiol Endocrinol Metab 2008;295(4):E868–75.
47. Suryawan A, Torrazza RM, Gazzaneo MC, et al. Enteral leucine supplementation increases protein synthesis in skeletal and cardiac muscles and visceral tissues of neonatal pigs through mTORC1-dependent pathways. Pediatr Res 2012; 71(4 Pt 1):324–31.
48. Belfort MB, Gillman MW, Buka SL, et al. Preterm infant linear growth and adiposity gain: trade-offs for later weight status and intelligence quotient. J Pediatr 2013;163(6):1564–9.
49. Forbes GB. Relation of lean body mass to height in children and adolescents. Pediatr Res 1972;6(1):32–7.
50. Kennaugh JM, Bell AW, Teng C, et al. Ontogenetic changes in the rates of protein synthesis and leucine oxidation during fetal life. Pediatr Res 1987;22(6):688–92.
51. Meier PR, Peterson RG, Bonds DR, et al. Rates of protein synthesis and turnover in fetal life. Am J Physiol 1981;240(3):E320–4.
52. Fomon SJ, Ziegler EE, Vazquez HD. Human milk and the small premature infant. Am J Dis Child 1977;131(4):463–7.
53. Ziegler EE, O'Donnell AM, Nelson SE, et al. Body composition of the reference fetus. Growth 1976;40(4):329–41.
54. Widdowson EM. The fetus and the newborn. In: Assail B, editor. Biology of gestation, vol. 2. New York: Academic Press; 1972. p. 1–44.
55. Ziegler EE. Meeting the nutritional needs of the low-birth-weight infant. Ann Nutr Metab 2011;58(Suppl 1):8–18.
56. Ziegler EE. Protein requirements of preterm infants. In: Fomon SJ, Heird WC, editors. Energy and protein needs during infancy. New York: Academic Press; 1986. p. 69–85.
57. Ziegler EE. Protein requirements of very low birth weight infants. J Pediatr Gastroenterol Nutr 2007;45(Suppl 3):S170–4.
58. Kashyap S, Forsyth M, Zucker C, et al. Effects of varying protein and energy intakes on growth and metabolic response in low birth weight infants. J Pediatr 1986;108(6):955–63.
59. Kashyap S, Schulze KF, Ramakrishnan R, et al. Evaluation of a mathematical model for predicting the relationship between protein and energy intakes of low-birth-weight infants and the rate and composition of weight gain. Pediatr Res 1994;35(6):704–12.
60. Fairey AK, Butte NF, Mehta N, et al. Nutrient accretion in preterm infants fed formula with different protein: energy ratios. J Pediatr Gastroenterol Nutr 1997; 25(1):37–45.

61. Cooke R, Embleton N, Rigo J, et al. High protein pre-term infant formula: effect on nutrient balance, metabolic status and growth. Pediatr Res 2006;59(2):265–70.

62. Cormack BE, Bloomfield FH, Dezoete A, et al. Does more protein in the first week of life change outcomes for very low birthweight babies? J Paediatr Child Health 2011;47(12):898–903.

63. Hanson C, Sundermeier J, Dugick L, et al. Implementation, process, and outcomes of nutrition best practices for infants <1500 g. Nutr Clin Pract 2011; 26(5):614–24.

64. Roggero P, Gianni ML, Orsi A, et al. Implementation of nutritional strategies decreases postnatal growth restriction in preterm infants. PLoS One 2012;7(12): e51166.

65. Hay WW Jr, Regnault TR, Brown LD. Fetal requirements and placental transfer of nitrogenous compounds. In: Polin RA, Fox WW, Abman SH, editors. Fetal and neonatal physiology. 4th edition. Philadelphia: Saunders, an imprint of Elsevier, Inc; 2011. p. 585–614.

66. Svenningsen NW, Lindroth M, Lindquist B. Growth in relation to protein intake of low birth weight infants. Early Hum Dev 1982;6(1):47–58.

67. Adams-Chapman I. Neurodevelopmental outcome of the late preterm infant. Clin Perinatol 2006;33(4):947–64.

68. Carlson SE. Feeding after discharge: growth, development, and long-term effects. In: Tsang RC, Uauy R, Koletzko B, et al, editors. Nutrition of the preterm infant: scientific basis and practical guidelines. 2nd edition. Cincinnati (OH): Digital Educational Publishing, Inc; 2005. p. 357–82.

69. Masor ML. Post discharge nutrition of the late preterm infant. EJ Neonatol Res 2012;2(2):101–2.

70. Cooke RJ, Griffin IJ, McCormick K. Adiposity is not altered in preterm infants fed with a nutrient-enriched formula after hospital discharge. Pediatr Res 2010; 67(6):660–4.

71. Pittaluga E, Vernal P, Llanos A, et al. Benefits of supplemented preterm formulas on insulin sensitivity and body composition after discharge from the neonatal intensive care unit. J Pediatr 2011;159(6):926–32.

72. Towers HM, Schulze KF, Ramakrishnan R, et al. Energy expended by low birth weight infants in the deposition of protein and fat. Pediatr Res 1997;41(4 Pt 1): 584–9.

73. van Goudoever JB, Sulkers EJ, Lafeber HN, et al. Short-term growth and substrate use in very-low-birth-weight infants fed formulas with different energy contents. Am J Clin Nutr 2000;71(3):816–21.

74. Micheli JL, Schutz Y. Protein. In: Tsang RC, Lucas A, Uauy R, et al, editors. Nutritional needs of the preterm infant. 1st edition. Pawling (NY): Caduceus Medical Publishers; 1993. p. 29–46.

75. Taroni F, Liotto N, Morlacchi L, et al. Body composition in small for gestational age newborns. Pediatr Med Chir 2008;30(6):296–301.

76. Brown LD, Hay WW Jr. The nutritional dilemma for preterm infants: how to promote neurocognitive development and linear growth, but reduce the risk of obesity. J Pediatr 2013;163(6):1543–5.

77. Moya F, Sisk PM, Walsh KR, et al. A new liquid human milk fortifier and linear growth in preterm infants. Pediatrics 2012;130(4):e928–35.

78. Avery ME, Clow CL, Menkes JH, et al. Transient tyrosinemia of the newborn: dietary and clinical aspects. Pediatrics 1967;39(3):378–84.

79. Mathews J, Partington MW. The plasma tyrosine levels of premature babies. Arch Dis Child 1964;39:371–8.

80. Snyderman SE, Holt LE Jr, Nortn PM, et al. The plasma aminogram. I. Influence of the level of protein intake and a comparison of whole protein and amino acid diets. Pediatr Res 1968;2(2):131–44.

81. Goldman HI, Freudenthal R, Holland B, et al. Clinical effects of two different levels of protein intake on low-birth-weight infants. J Pediatr 1969;74(6):881–9.

82. Goldman HI, Liebman OB, Freudenthal R, et al. Effects of early dietary protein intake on low-birth-weight infants: evaluation at 3 years of age. J Pediatr 1971;78(1):126–9.

83. Goldman HI, Goldman J, Kaufman I, et al. Late effects of early dietary protein intake on low-birth-weight infants. J Pediatr 1974;85(6):764–9.

84. Kashyap S. Enteral intake for very low birth weight infants: what should the composition be? Semin Perinatol 2007;31(2):74–82.

85. Cibulskis CC, Bowles M. Metabolic acidosis associated with liquid acidified human milk fortifier. AAP Section on Perinatal Pediatrics Scientific and Educational Program. 2013. Ref type: Abstract. AAP National Conference and Exhibition, Orlando, Florida, October 25–27, 2013.

86. Thoene M, Hanson C, Lyden E, et al. Comparison of the effect of two human milk fortifiers on clinical outcomes in premature infants. Nutrients 2014;6:261–75.

87. Bhatia J, Rassin DK, Cerreto MC, et al. Effect of protein/energy ratio on growth and behavior of premature infants: preliminary findings. J Pediatr 1991;119(1 Pt 1):103–10.

88. Cooke RJ, Watson D, Werkman S, et al. Effects of type of dietary protein on acid-base status, protein nutritional status, plasma levels of amino acids, and nutrient balance in the very low birth weight infant. J Pediatr 1992;121(3):444–51.

89. Moro G, Minoli I, Boehm G, et al. Postprandial plasma amino acids in preterm infants: influence of the protein source. Acta Paediatr 1999;88(8):885–9.

90. Rivera A Jr, Bell EF, Bier DM. Effect of intravenous amino acids on protein metabolism of preterm infants during the first three days of life. Pediatr Res 1993;33(2):106–11.

91. van Goudoever JB, Colen T, Wattimena JL, et al. Immediate commencement of amino acid supplementation in preterm infants: effect on serum amino acid concentrations and protein kinetics on the first day of life. J Pediatr 1995;127(3):458–65.

92. van Lingen RA, van Goudoever JB, Luijendijk IH, et al. Effects of early amino acid administration during total parenteral nutrition on protein metabolism in pre-term infants. Clin Sci (Lond) 1992;82(2):199–203.

93. Ridout E, Melara D, Rottinghaus S, et al. Blood urea nitrogen concentration as a marker of amino-acid intolerance in neonates with birthweight less than 1250 g. J Perinatol 2005;25(2):130–3.

94. Tchirikov M, Schroder HJ, Hecher K. Ductus venosus shunting in the fetal venous circulation: regulatory mechanisms, diagnostic methods and medical importance. Ultrasound Obstet Gynecol 2006;27(4):452–61.

95. Yajnik CS. Obesity epidemic in India: intrauterine origins? Proc Nutr Soc 2004;63(3):387–96.

96. Lapillonne A, Braillon P, Claris O, et al. Body composition in appropriate and in small for gestational age infants. Acta Paediatr 1997;86(2):196–200.

97. Padoan A, Rigano S, Ferrazzi E, et al. Differences in fat and lean mass proportions in normal and growth-restricted fetuses. Am J Obstet Gynecol 2004;191(4):1459–64.

98. Tudehope D, Vento M, Bhutta Z, et al. Nutritional requirements and feeding recommendations for small for gestational age infants. J Pediatr 2013;162(Suppl 3):S81–9.

99. De Jesus LC, Pappas A, Shankaran S, et al. Outcomes of small for gestational age infants born at <27 weeks' gestation. J Pediatr 2013;163(1):55–60.

100. Ong KK. Catch-up growth in small for gestational age babies: good or bad? Curr Opin Endocrinol Diabetes Obes 2007;14(1):30–4.

101. Boehm G, Senger H, Muller D, et al. Metabolic differences between AGA- and SGA-infants of very low birthweight. II. Relationship to protein intake. Acta Paediatr Scand 1988;77(5):642–6.

102. Morley R, Fewtrell MS, Abbott RA, et al. Neurodevelopment in children born small for gestational age: a randomized trial of nutrient-enriched versus standard formula and comparison with a reference breastfed group. Pediatrics 2004;113(3 Pt 1):515–21.

103. Bellotti M, Pennati G, De Gasperi C, et al. Simultaneous measurements of umbilical venous, fetal hepatic, and ductus venosus blood flow in growth-restricted human fetuses. Am J Obstet Gynecol 2004;190(5):1347–58.

104. Kunz C, Lonnerdal B. Re-evaluation of the whey protein/casein ratio of human milk. Acta Paediatr 1992;81(2):107–12.

105. Benson J, Neylan M, Masor ML, et al. Approaches and considerations in determining the protein and amino acid composition of term and preterm infant formula. Int Dairy J 1998;8:405–12.

106. Gaull GE, Rassin DK, Raiha NC, et al. Milk protein quantity and quality in low-birth-weight infants. III. Effects on sulfur amino acids in plasma and urine. J Pediatr 1977;90(3):348–55.

107. Raiha NC, Heinonen K, Rassin DK, et al. Milk protein quantity and quality in low-birthweight infants: I. metabolic responses and effects on growth. Pediatrics 1976;57(5):659–84.

108. Rassin DK, Gaull GE, Heinonen K, et al. Milk protein quantity and quality in low-birth-weight infants: II. Effects on selected aliphatic amino acids in plasma and urine. Pediatrics 1977;59(3):407–22.

109. Rassin DK, Gaull GE, Raiha NC, et al. Milk protein quantity and quality in low-birth-weight infants. IV. Effects on tyrosine and phenylalanine in plasma and urine. J Pediatr 1977;90(3):356–60.

110. Rassin DK, Sturman JA, Guall GE. Taurine and other free amino acids in milk of man and other mammals. Early Hum Dev 1978;2(1):1–13.

111. Schreiner RL, Brady MS, Ernst JA, et al. Lack of lactobezoars in infants given predominantly whey protein formulas. Am J Dis Child 1982;136(5):437–9.

112. Boirie Y, Dangin M, Gachon P, et al. Slow and fast dietary proteins differently modulate postprandial protein accretion. Proc Natl Acad Sci U S A 1997; 94(26):14930–5.

113. El-Kadi SW, Suryawan A, Gazzaneo MC, et al. Anabolic signaling and protein deposition are enhanced by intermittent compared with continuous feeding in skeletal muscle of neonates. Am J Physiol Endocrinol Metab 2012;302(6): E674–86.

114. El-Kadi SW, Gazzaneo MC, Suryawan A, et al. Viscera and muscle protein synthesis in neonatal pigs is increased more by intermittent bolus than by continuous feeding. Pediatr Res 2013;74(2):154–62.

115. Boutry C, El-Kadi SW, Suryawan A, et al. Leucine pulses enhance skeletal muscle protein synthesis during continuous feeding in neonatal pigs. Am J Physiol Endocrinol Metab 2013;305(5):E620–31.

116. Schanler RJ, Shulman RJ, Lau C, et al. Feeding strategies for premature infants: randomized trial of gastrointestinal priming and tube-feeding method. Pediatrics 1999;103(2):434–9.

117. Maggio L, Zuppa AA, Sawatzki G, et al. Higher urinary excretion of essential amino acids in preterm infants fed protein hydrolysates. Acta Paediatr 2005; 94(1):75–84.
118. Rigo J, Salle BL, Picaud JC, et al. Nutritional evaluation of protein hydrolysate formulas. Eur J Clin Nutr 1995;49(Suppl 1):S26–38.
119. Agostoni C, Buonocore G, Carnielli VP, et al. Enteral nutrient supply for preterm infants: commentary from the European Society of Paediatric Gastroenterology, Hepatology and Nutrition Committee on Nutrition. J Pediatr Gastroenterol Nutr 2010;50(1):85–91.
120. Nutrient needs and feeding of premature infants. Nutrition Committee, Canadian Paediatric Society. CMAJ 1995;152(11):1765–85.
121. American Academy of Pediatrics Committee on Nutrition. Nutritional needs of preterm infants. In: Kleinman RE, editor. Pediatric nutrition handbook American Academy of Pediatrics. 1st edition. Elk Grove Village (IL): American Academy of Pediatrics; 2013. p. 23–54.
122. Klein CJ. Nutrient requirements for preterm infant formulas. J Nutr 2002; 132(6 Suppl 1):1395S–577S.

Fortification of Human Milk in Very Low Birth Weight Infants (VLBW <1500 g Birth Weight)

David H. Adamkin, MD[a], Paula G. Radmacher, MSPH, PhD[b],*

KEYWORDS

- Very low birth weight infants • Preterm human milk • Human milk fortification
- Necrotizing enterocolitis • Postnatal growth restriction • Neurodevelopment

KEY POINTS

- Human milk is the preferred feeding for all infants.
- Preterm human milk has immunologic and neurodevelopmental benefits for very-low-birth-weight and extremely low-birth-weight infants that persist beyond the neonatal intensive care unit hospitalization.
- Preterm human milk is nutritionally inadequate, especially in protein, to fully support the growth needs of the very-low-birth-weight and extremely low-birth-weight infant.
- Several products and strategies are available to fortify preterm human milk.
- Human milk analyzers can be used to gain information about nutrient content before adding fortifiers.

INTRODUCTION

The American Academy of Pediatrics supports the feeding of human milk for all infants, term and preterm.[1] The benefits of human milk over formula feedings include nutritional, immunologic, developmental, psychological, social, and economic advantages. In the short term, feeding human milk to very-low-birth-weight (VLBW) infants has been associated with reductions in morbidity and mortality specifically related to sepsis and necrotizing enterocolitis (NEC).[2–7] Long-term beneficial effects of human milk for extremely low-birth-weight infants (<1000 g) in the neonatal intensive care unit (NICU) have also been shown from data from the Eunice Kennedy Shriver National

a Division of Neonatal Medicine, Department of Pediatrics, University of Louisville School of Medicine, 571 South Floyd Street, Suite 342, Louisville, KY 40202-3830, USA; b Neonatal Nutrition Research Laboratory, Department of Pediatrics, University of Louisville School of Medicine, 511 South Floyd Street, Room 107, Louisville, KY 40202, USA
* Corresponding author.
E-mail address: paula.radmacher@louisville.edu

Clin Perinatol 41 (2014) 405–421
http://dx.doi.org/10.1016/j.clp.2014.02.010
0095-5108/14/$ – see front matter © 2014 Elsevier Inc. All rights reserved.

Institute of Child Health and Development Neonatal Research Network.[8] Nutrition data collected on 773 such infants showed positive effects related to human milk intake in developmental outcomes at 18 months of age. At 30 months, increased receipt of human milk during NICU hospitalization was associated with higher Bayley Mental Developmental Index (MDI) scores, higher Bayley behavior score percentiles for emotional regulation, and fewer hospitalizations between discharge and 30 months.[8] For each 10 mL/k/d increase in receipt of human milk, the MDI increased 0.59 points. This persistence of effect far beyond the neonatal period, through 30 months of age, in extremely premature infants provides evidence that providing mother's milk to VLBW infants should be a priority in the NICU and after discharge.

In addition, infants receiving their mother's milk show

- Improved gastrointestinal function, digestion, and absorption of nutrients[9]
- Improved cognitive[10–12] and visual development[11,13]
- Improved host defense with reduced rates of infection (sepsis, NEC, and urinary tract infection)[14,15]
- Less respiratory illness[11]
- Enhanced maternal psychological well-being and maternal-infant bonding[1]
- More rapid attainment of full enteral feeding and shorter duration of hospitalization[9]

However, there are nutritional limitations of human milk for these vulnerable infants that must be addressed.

PRETERM AND DONOR HUMAN MILK

There are challenges in trying to provide exclusive human milk feedings for the VLBW infant and to meet nutritional requirements: inadequate milk supply of the mother, the high variability in nutrient content of the milk itself,[16–19] clinically necessary volume restriction in some infants, and the nutrient limitations of the milk itself. Human milk composition is known to vary with volume and method of milk expression, the time of day, the type of milk obtained (foremilk or hindmilk), and the stage of lactation.[20–23] There may be 2-fold to 3-fold differences in protein and fat (energy) regardless of the stage of lactation simply because of these factors (**Fig. 1**).[16,24,25]

In the latest recommendation from the American Academy of Pediatrics Committee on Breastfeeding Medicine, donor human milk (DHM) should be used when mother's milk is unavailable.[1] DHM is generally term in quality and has been pasteurized to reduce the risk of infection. Pasteurization decreases the activity of many bioactive factors that have roles in protecting the infant from infection and preparing the gastrointestinal system for extrauterine life.[26–30] In addition, the processing of DHM (thawing, pooling, pouring into new containers, and so on) most likely decreases fat and protein.[31] Thus, although DHM is preferable to bovine-based formula as a substitute for preterm human milk (PHM), both are inadequate to meet the nutritional needs of the VLBW infant without multicomponent fortification.[18] Until recently, those fortifier products have been derived from cow milk–based products, which may reduce the beneficial effects of human milk administration.

When VLBW infants receive insufficient amounts of nutrients, poor growth is ultimately observed and is a surrogate for inadequate nutrition. Slow growth because of inadequate nutrition is associated with poor neurocognitive outcome.[32,33] Substantial evidence suggests that it is mainly inadequate intake of protein that is responsible for these outcomes.[32,34–36] Although energy is important, it plays much less of a role as a cause of slow growth. Although the exact requirements of vitamins, minerals, and

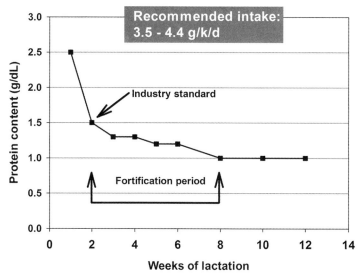

Fig. 1. Preterm human milk protein content during 12 weeks of lactation and fortification. (*Data from* Schanler RJ, Oh W. Composition of breast milk obtained from mothers of premature infants as compared to breast milk obtained from donors. J Pediatr 1980;96(4):679–81.)

micronutrients for preterm infants are not exactly known, they are not normally problematic, although there are occasional reports of deficiencies.[37,38] Modest shortfalls or excesses of these nutrients do not seem to cause problems.[39]

MACRONUTRIENT REQUIREMENTS OF THE VLBW INFANT

Because the neonatal period represents a critical time in which the brain is especially vulnerable to nutritional deficits, attention to the details of nutritional management is critical. Neither insufficiency nor excess is desirable. The specific deficits (primarily protein) of both PHM and DHM must be addressed with products that bring them in line with recommended intakes for protein and energy. **Table 1** shows protein and protein/energy ratio recommendations based on epochs of postmenstrual age and the need for catch-up growth.[40]

Protein is limiting for growth and is essential for optimal neurodevelopment.[41] Appropriate protein fortification of human milk is therefore critical. Although there has been concern that too much enteral protein is unhealthy, more recent data on requirements

Table 1
Advisable protein recommendation for growing preterm infants needing catch-up growth

Postmenstrual Age (wk)	With Need for Catch-Up (g/k/d)	Protein/Energy
26–30	4.4	3.4
30–36	3.8–4.2	3.3
36–40	3.0–3.4	2.6–2.8

Data from Rigo J. Protein, amino acid and other nitrogen compounds. In: Tsang RC, Uauy R, Koletzko B, et al, editors. Nutrition of the preterm infant: scientific basis and practical guidelines. 2nd edition. Cincinnati (OH): Digital Educational Publishing, Inc; 2005. p. 45.

have shown that VLBW infants require more protein than previously thought and that there is a wide range of safety with current products and approaches.[39,41–43]

GOALS OF FORTIFICATION

The primary goal of any nutritional regimen for VLBW infants is to support a postnatal growth rate that is similar to the intrauterine growth rate (15 g/k/d) with appropriate body composition. To achieve that goal, there must be an adequate balance between protein and energy (see **Table 1**). As the understanding of nutrient needs for VLBW infants advances, products and processes have begun to adapt.

FORTIFICATION PRODUCTS

With the goal of providing preterm infants with enteral protein in the range of 3.5 to 4.5 g/k/d to support their rapid growth, current options for fortifying PHM are more varied than ever before (**Table 2**). The Centers for Disease Control and Prevention no longer recommend powder formulas and human milk fortifiers for preterm infants because of the risk of bacterial contamination and subsequent bacteremia.[44,45]

For women that have insufficient milk supply, 30 kcal/oz preterm formulas (PTF30) have been used to increase the protein and to extend her limited supply. However, for the woman that is producing adequate amounts of milk to meet her infant's needs, using PTF30 as a fortifier displaces a substantial volume of PHM. The infant also receives significant bovine antigen with each feeding, which may dilute the benefits that PHM provides. Concentrated fortifiers increase the protein without the additional amount of fat and carbohydrate that would be provided in PTF30.

The Enfamil Human Milk Fortifier Acidified Liquid (HMF-AL; Mead Johnson Nutrition, Evansville, IN, USA) provides the highest amount of protein of the bovine fortifiers (2.2 g in 4 vials added to 100 mL PHM). As a concentrated liquid, it displaces less PHM than PTF30 and delivers less bovine antigen. However, it is possible that protein concentrations in milk fortified with HMF-AL could exceed 5 g/k/d if the mother is producing milk with higher than expected protein (>1.5 g/dL). If milk analysis is available, the number of vials added to the mother's milk may be adjusted so that the final profile meets the desired targets without exceeding them (**Fig. 2**).

Moya and colleagues[46] reported a study in which infants received PHM fortified with either the HMF-AL (5 vials) or a powder fortifier (4 packets) per 100 mL. Infants receiving the HMF-AL showed significantly better gains in weight and head circumference at day 28 compared with infants receiving powder-fortified PHM. There were no significant differences between groups in proportions of infants with abnormal laboratory values, including pH and Pco_2.

Erickson and colleagues[47] created an in vitro simulation of acidified human milk using citric acid in place of the HMF-AL. Split samples of human milk were either acidified to a pH ~4.5 or left untreated. The investigators noted a significant decrease in white cell content, total protein, and lipase activity in the treated samples compared with the untreated samples. The clinical meaning of these changes is unknown but the authors suggest that these effects may not be beneficial for the preterm infant.

Similac Human Milk Fortifier (Abbott Nutrition, Columbus, OH, USA), mixed as 4 vials plus 100 mL PHM, provides an additional 1.4 g protein. In its concentrated form, it displaces less milk than PTF30 but provides less added protein than HMF-AL. At the prescribed proportions, it is unlikely to meet recommendations (3.5–4.5 g/k/d of protein) with DHM or PHM with lower protein content.

Similac Liquid Protein additive is a sterile liquid that can boost protein content (1 g/6 mL) in a PHM or PHM-fortifier mixture. When using PHM produced beyond

Table 2
Fortifier products

Product	Enfamil[a]		Similac[b]			Prolacta[c]			
	Human Milk Fortifier- Acidified Liquid	Premature 30	Special Care 30	Human Milk Fortifier	Liquid Protein	+4 H² HMF[c]	+6 H² HMF[c]	+8 H² HMF[c]	+10 H² HMF[c]
Unit volume (mL)	5	As needed	As needed	5	6	20	30	40	100
Mixing ratio	4 vials + 100 mL PHM	75 mL + 100 mL PHM	75 mL + 100 mL PHM	4 vials + 100 mL PHM	As needed	20 mL + 80 mL PHM	30 mL + 70 mL PHM	60 mL + 40 mL PHM	50 mL + 50 mL PHM
Nutrients added to native human milk									
Calories (kcal)	30	75	76	14	4	28	42	56	71
Protein (g)	2.2	2.27	2.28	1.0	1	1.2	1.8	2.4	3.0
Fat (g)	2.3	3.9	5.0	0.4	0	1.8	2.8	3.6	4.6
Carbohydrate (g)	<1.2 per vial	8.3	5.9	1.8	0	1.8	2.7	3.6	4.5

Abbreviation: PHM, Preterm human milk.
[a] Mead Johnson Nutrition, Evansville, IN.
[b] Abbott Nutrition, Columbus, OH.
[c] Prolacta Bioscience, Monrovia, CA. The nutrient values provided are for general reference only. They are based on target values and averages for Prolact + H² HMF.

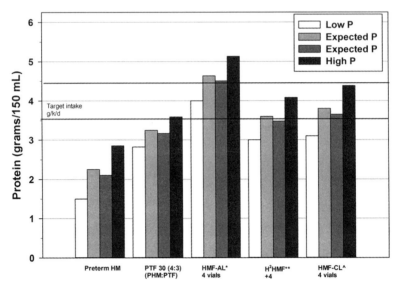

Fig. 2. Preterm human milk protein (g) achieved with 4 different fortifiers when fed at 150 mL. * Mead Johnson Nutrition. ** Prolacta. ^ Abbott Nutrition. (*Data from* Radmacher PG, Lewis SL, Adamkin D. Individualizing fortification of human milk using real time human milk analysis. J Neonatal Perinatal Med 2013;6:319–23.)

4 to 6 weeks or DHM, it is likely that protein will be more similar to term milk and be inadequate for the growth needs of the VLBW infant. Liquid protein may be added in conjunction with fortifier if the protein content of the native milk is especially low. This product is designed to be an additive, not a sole nutrition source. It is supplied in a 54-mL bottle that contains a total of 9 g of protein. Leftover product must be refrigerated after opening and used within 24 hours or discarded.

The ProlactPlus products (Prolacta Bioscience, Monrovia, CA, USA) are unique in that they are concentrated human milk products. They are created in a variety of additive concentrations (+4, +6, +8, +10 kcal/oz) to provide the clinician with flexibility in constructing an all-human milk feeding that can address specific issues, such as fluid restriction, and still provide adequate protein and energy for growth (see **Table 2**). The ProlactPlus products also supplement electrolytes and minerals. The benefits of an exclusive HM diet in reducing NEC are discussed elsewhere.

APPROACHES TO FORTIFICATION

There are 3 approaches one can take to fortifying PHM:

- Standard, fixed dosage enhancement of the preterm or DHM
- Adjustable fortification using a surrogate for protein nutriture to modify the dosage of fortification
- Targeted (customized, individualized) fortification or fortification triggered by poor growth and results from human milk analysis (HMA)

STANDARD FORTIFICATION

The most common strategy for fortification of human milk assumes an average composition of human milk (native milk) at about 2 weeks of lactation (1.5 g/dL) and then adds a fixed dosage of fortifier (standard, fixed dosage) (**Fig. 1**). This method does not take into account that the caloric and nutrient content of the milk varies between mothers, duration of lactation, and even individual samples from the same mother.[5,16,24,48] The resulting milk probably contains less protein and energy than one would assume.

A recent *Cochrane Review* selected 13 trials that randomized (or quasi-randomized) allocation to supplementation of PHM with multiple nutrients or no supplementation.[49] Multicomponent fortification was associated with short-term increases in weight gain, linear growth, and head circumference. Nitrogen retention and blood urea levels appeared to be increased. It was not clear if there was an effect on bone mineralization itself. There were insufficient data to evaluate long-term neurodevelopmental and growth outcomes in these studies, although there appeared to be no effect on growth beyond 1 year.

Despite fortification, studies have shown that preterm infants fed fortified PHM continue to grow more slowly than infants fed preterm formula.[34,43,50,51] Henriksen and colleagues[52] conducted a study of 127 VLBW infants fed primarily fortified PHM, evaluating nutrient intake and other relevant factors associated with extrauterine growth restriction (body weight <10th percentile at discharge). Infants were fed their own mother's milk or DHM that was fortified when enteral intake reached 120 mL/k/d. They demonstrated that 58% of these infants were growth restricted at discharge. The recommended energy and nutrient intakes for growing VLBW infants were not achieved.

Recent studies have shown that the protein content of expressed human milk is often lower than the assumed 1.5 g/dL[41,42] and with standard fortification would deliver inadequate amounts of protein for the VLBW infant.[19] As mentioned above, banked DHM, which is most often provided by mothers of term infants, is likely to have an even lower protein content[18] and requires more than standard fortification to compensate. Because of concerns about the consequences of "high-protein" intakes in these infants, commercial producers of HM fortifiers have chosen to design their products for milk with a modest protein content (1.5 g/dL, representing milk produced at 2–3 weeks) (**Fig. 1**). Therefore, even when the milk protein content is at the higher end of the possible range of protein content, the clinician is essentially guaranteed that protein intake would never be "too high." **Table 3** shows data that compare

Table 3
Macronutrient analysis results (mean ± SD)

	Stage of Lactation			Donor Human Milk (term)	P
	0–2 wk	2–4 wk	≥4 wk		
Protein (g/dL)	1.7 ± 0.3	1.5 ± 0.2	1.3 ± 0.4	1.0 ± 0.1	<.02 (DHM vs
Range	1.3–2.8	1.2–2.0	0.9–1.9	0.8–1.1	PHM all stages)
Fat (g/dL)	3.0 ± 0.9	3.6 ± 1.1	3.8 ± 0.9	2.5 ± 0.3	≤.015 (DHM vs PHM
Range	1.0–5.7	1.8–6.2	2.1–5.5	2.2–3.0	0–2 wk and ≥4 wk)
Lactose (g/dL)	6.5 ± 0.5	6.6 ± 0.3	6.5 ± 0.2	6.1 ± 0.4	<.005 (DHM vs
Range	5.1–7.9	6.4–7.5	5.9–7.1	5.5–6.7	PHM all stages)
Energy (kcal/oz)	17.2 ± 2.4	18.6 ± 2.9	18.9 ± 2.6	14.6 ± 1.4	.021 (DHM vs PHM
Range	12.4–24.5	13.6–25.7	14.2–23.6	13.1–16.6	0–2 wk and ≥4 wk)

Abbreviations: DHM, Donor human milk; PHM, Preterm human milk.
Data from Radmacher PG, Lewis SL, Adamkin D. Individualizing fortification of human milk using real time human milk analysis. J Neonatal Perinatal Med 2013;6:319–23.

human milk macronutrient profiles over 3 separate 2-week periods of lactation to DHM obtained from a milk bank.[53] The expected decline in protein is observed and protein concentrations are statistically higher than that in DHM at every time point measured. The difference in lactose is statistically significant but not clinically relevant.[53] Mean energy is less than the "assumed" 20 kcal/oz and varies widely. Energy content in DHM is the lowest of all.

ADJUSTABLE FORTIFICATION

Adjustable fortification is an approach centered on the VLBW infant's metabolic response to enteral protein intake. The amount of added fortifier (protein) is based on changes in serial blood urea nitrogen (BUN) measurements and assumes that BUN is the appropriate surrogate for adequate protein nutriture. In essence, this method looks to the infant to indicate a need for more (or less) protein by an increasing, decreasing, or static BUN response to enteral feedings. If this assumption is correct, excessive protein intake should be avoided. It does not require the technology and labor to conduct serial analyses of milk samples and it represents a potentially practical method for managing the routine fortification of human milk.

This method was developed for a study comparing standard fortification (4 packets + 100 mL PHM or DHM) with an adjustable regimen in which fortifier and/ or protein was added or subtracted from fortified PHM based on changes in serum BUN using a target of 9 to 14 mg/dL.[54] This study included 32 preterm infants between 600 and 1760 g birth weight. Infants were on their assigned regimens for 3 weeks, receiving 60% of their volume of HM from their own mothers' milk and 40% from DHM. Nutrient intakes were calculated for these infants using assumed macronutrient values and applied to the intake volume. For those in the adjustable arm, any changes in the amount of fortifier and/or protein powder added to the native HM were included in the final calculations. Groups were thought to be receiving comparable intakes of fat and energy, with protein increased in the infants in the adjustable arm of the study. Body weight and head circumference gains averaged 14 g/k/d and 0.7 cm/week (standard) compared with 18 g/k/d and 1.0 cm/week (adjustable) ($P<0.01$ for weight and <0.05 for head circumference, respectively, between groups).

In a follow-up to this study, the investigators reported the actual nutrient content of the milks used in the previous study compared with their calculated values.[41] The assumed values for both groups were substantially lower than expected for protein. Protein content of PHM decreases as lactation continues and is likely responsible for the poor postnatal growth of infants with standard fortification.

The results of their study suggest that simply increasing the amount of fortifier can be an approach for adding more protein. The assumed protein intake for infants fed their own mother's milk or banked milk was greater than the actual intake because of inaccurate estimates of protein content in the native milk. The result was that infants received as much as 0.6 to 0.8 g/k/d less protein than expected. This is a significant discrepancy that could affect growth. Another consideration is that fortifiers are multi-nutrient products. For the purpose of protein enrichment of PHM, additional fortifier increases not only the protein but also all of the other nutrients found in the products (vitamins, minerals, fats, carbohydrate), which may not be desirable.

In a 2009 editorial about the adjustable fortification study, William Hay Jr. asks the question, "would an additional 1 g/k/d of protein be too much for those infants in whom the mother has good milk protein content?"[55] He concludes that it is not likely. Many reports of human milk protein content consistently show levels in mothers' milk for preterm infants to be well under 2 g/dL.[56–58] Adding 1 g/k/d of protein to such milk would produce no more than 3 g/dL and an intake of less than 4.5 g/k/d at 150 mL/k/d. Also, the total protein intake would decrease as the duration of lactation progresses and protein content of the native milk naturally decreases.

TARGETED FORTIFICATION

Traditional milk analysis using reference chemical analysis, which is laborious, time-consuming, and not available in real-time, has given way to infrared spectroscopy.[57,59,60] These devices provide results quickly, are easy to use, and are becoming more common for real-time nutrient analysis of human milk (see section on technology). Information from these analyses enables the nutrition support team to more specifically individualize fortification for any preterm infant. These devices are not generally available for routine clinical use.

The third strategy in human milk fortification for VLBW infants is targeted fortification in which the native milk is analyzed for macronutrient content and then fortified in such a way as to reach the desired targets. This method was studied more than 10 years ago using mid-infrared (MIR) spectroscopy to analyze macronutrients in human milk.[58] Using the results as a guide to individualized fortification, the study aimed to meet a protein target of 3.5 g/k/d. Ultimately, the protein intake was slightly less than desired but infants grew at ~15 g/k/d and had acceptable head circumference growth.

Rochow and colleagues[57] reported their experience with establishing an infrastructure to perform target fortification of breast milk safely in the NICU by measuring and adjusting for fat, protein, and carbohydrate content on a daily basis. Twelve-hour pools of human milk for 10 prospectively enrolled infants were analyzed by near-infrared spectroscopy (NIR; SpectraStar, Unity Scientific, Brookfield, CT, USA) and fortified to meet macronutrient recommendations from ESPGHAN.[61] Growth patterns were compared with similar historic controls. There were 650 pooled milk samples analyzed; all of them required at least 1 macronutrient adjustment. Milk osmolalities were checked for acceptability (400–480 mOsm/kg) to preclude preparation errors. Serum biochemistries from the infants all fell within expected ranges. When compared with historic controls, infants receiving targeted fortification grew at similar rates, ~20 g/k/d. There was a linear correlation between growth and milk intake among the targeted cohort ($R^2 = 0.68$), which was not seen in the matched controls. Rochow and colleagues suggest that the analytical approach allowed them to compensate for the variable composition of the native milk.

Radmacher and colleagues analyzed 83 discrete samples of human milk using MIR spectrophotometry (Calais Human Milk Analyzer; North American Instruments, Murrieta, CA, USA).[53] Analyses confirmed that across lactation periods (0–2 weeks, 2–4 weeks, and >4 weeks) protein declined as expected with DHM having the lowest protein content (see **Table 3**). From those samples, 3 PHM profiles were chosen, as well as a representative sample of DHM, to then calculate the nutrient content of those samples if they were fortified in the usual manner with a variety of products and fed at 150 mL/k/d. Milk profiles were chosen to represent expected protein and energy, expected protein but increased energy, high protein and marginal energy, and low protein with low energy (DHM). **Fig. 2** shows the calculated protein content for these samples. As expected, all unfortified milk samples failed to meet recommendations for the VLBW infant. Examining the various fortification strategies, one can see that the macronutrient profile of the native milk has a substantial influence on the resulting fortified feeding. For low protein milks (DHM or milk from women that are several weeks into lactation) or milks that have more protein than expected, alternative fortification algorithms can be implemented to adjust protein content (**Fig. 3**). Not all of these samples resulted in milks that would deliver 120 kcal/k/d, but in the presence of sufficient protein, energy is not growth limiting as long as it is in the range of 90 to 100 kcal/k.[41]

Radmacher and colleagues also evaluated their own fortification strategies by examining serum BUN before and during HM fortification.[56] In a study including 24 VLBW infants, pooled samples of PHM or DHM were analyzed (volume sufficient for a 24-h period) before adding 30 kcal PTF (4 parts HM + 3 parts PTF; Similac Special Care 30; Abbott Nutrition) or concentrated fortifier (4 vials + 100 mL HM; Enfamil Human Milk Fortifier Acidifed Liquid; Mead Johnson Nutrition). Milk was analyzed 1 to 2 times weekly and used to calculate the protein and energy content after fortifier was added. Serum BUN and growth data were collected from the week before fortification for an additional 4 weeks or until hospital discharge. Mean energy of the unfortified milk was ~17 kcal/oz and the protein content was ~1.4 g/dL. Infants receiving PHM fortified with HMF-AL received significantly more protein than infants receiving milk fortified with PTF30, although weight and head circumference gains were not statistically significantly different at any time. By the fourth week of fortification mean weight gain was ~16 g/k/d and head circumference growth was 0.8 to 0.9 cm/week. The mean BUN decreased significantly from approximately 17 mg/dL before fortification, as total parenteral nutrition was weaning off, to approximately 6 mg/dL after 1 week of fortification and even lower by the fourth week of fortification at 3.6 mg/dL.

It appears from this study that energy (90–115 kcal/k/d) was not growth limiting, in that the infants actually grew a bit more than fetal rate. BUN values were modest, even low, in this group of infants who were experiencing acceptable growth. Thus with the

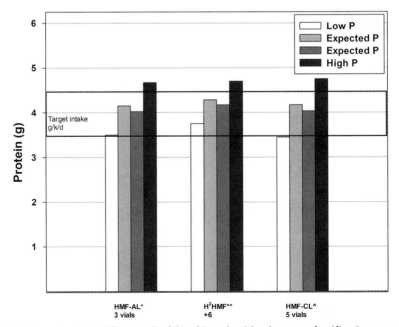

Fig. 3. Preterm human milk protein (g) achieved with alternate fortification strategies when fed at 150 mL. * Mead Johnson Nutrition. ** Prolacta. ^ Abbott Nutrition. (*Data from* Radmacher PG, Lewis SL, Adamkin D. Individualizing fortification of human milk using real time human milk analysis. J Neonatal Perinatal Med 2013;6:319–23.)

adjustable fortification strategy, more fortifier or other nutrients would have been added to the milk when, indeed, it was probably not warranted.

Although routine HM analysis is not readily available in most nurseries, infants showing slow growth (<15 g/k/d) or growth deceleration probably need more protein. The addition of 1 g/k/d of protein is a reasonable approach.[55]

TECHNOLOGY IN HM ANALYSIS

Currently available technology for HMA generally falls into 2 types: NIR and MIR spectroscopy (see **Table 4**). Each has been used in the dairy industry to monitor milk quality from multiple mammalian species with appropriate calibrations for the matrix being measured. These calibrations are based on results from well-accepted basic laboratory analyses, which are used to develop the computer models that convert the spectrometric data into quantitative results. Adaptation of these instruments for analysis of human milk requires that calibrations be conducted with human milk in a similar manner.

Laboratory analysis of human milk for calibration purposes relies on well-accepted methods for protein, lactose, and fat.[62] Split samples of human milk are subjected to laboratory and instrument analysis for each macronutrient. The computer model is then adjusted based on these paired results to provide quantitative values for each macronutrient.

MIR transmission spectroscopy is the Association of Analytic Communities' (AOAC) certified method used in the dairy industry for milk macronutrient analysis.[62] The instrumentation includes a light source with filters that allow the transmission of specific wavelengths through a cuvette or flow cell, and a detector. Vibrations in the MIR spectrum are associated with defined functional groups, which directly correlate to fat, and lactose.[63–66] The transmitted values are converted to concentrations by the specific calibration models for each macronutrient. Energy content is calculated based on accepted values of 9 kcal/g for fat and 4 kcal/g each for protein and carbohydrate.

Casadio and colleagues[65] evaluated the accuracy and suitability of an MIR human milk analyzer for routine macronutrient analysis (Miris AB, Uppsala, Sweden). Using milk from term and preterm mothers at various stages of lactation, samples were tested in the laboratory and by a human milk analyzer in their native state as well as in dilution and altered states of skim and concentrated milk components. Although they found some statistically significant differences between laboratory and HMA results, they concluded that the differences could be explained by chemical principles in the laboratory methods and that they were "small in relation to the variation in the macronutrient concentrations reported for human milk" and "not clinically significant

Table 4	
Currently available human milk analyzers	
	Vendors
Calais Human Milk Analyzer[a] Mid-infrared	North American Instruments, Murrieta, CA, USA
SpectraStar Near-infrared	Unity Scientific, Columbia, MD, USA
Miris[b] Mid-infrared	Miris Holding AB, Uppsala, Sweden

[a] Currently undergoing FDA review for approval as a medical device.
[b] Not available in the United States.

in relation to the macronutrient intake for preterm infants." Their conclusion was that HMA was efficient and practical for use in the nutritional management of preterm infants being fed HM.

O'Neill and colleagues[59] conducted a similar study in which they tested samples by both laboratory and MIR analysis (Calais Human Milk Analyzer; North American Instruments) as part of a comparison with creamatocrit. Although creamatocrit analysis overestimated fat, and consequently energy, MIR and laboratory results for fat and energy were within 1%.

NIR devices have also been used to analyze macronutrients in human milk.[60,67] Although it is not the AOAC-approved method, NIR has been evaluated in a manner similar to the MIR device. Sauer and Kim[60] and Corvaglia and colleagues[67] compared NIR device results (SpectraStar; Unity Scientific and Fenir; Esetek Instruments, Rome, Italy, respectively) with laboratory-based analyses. Both teams found acceptable agreement between laboratory and analyzer results for protein, lactose, and fat.

Regardless of which device is used to analyze human milk samples, the inter-woman and intra-woman variability of human milk has been reinforced in several recent studies.[42,53,57,60] It is clear that the assumption of 20 kcal/oz and 1.5 g/dL protein is inaccurate for a large number of women who are expressing milk for their preterm infants. As nutritional adequacy in support of rapid growth and brain development is extremely important during this critical period when VLBW infants are in the NICU, data from periodic HM analysis can augment the overall nutritional support plan. As more institutions acquire this technology and report their findings, nurseries that do not have it may benefit from others' experiences.

EXCLUSIVE HUMAN MILK FEEDING FOR PREVENTION OF NEC

NEC is the most significant gastrointestinal emergency occurring among VLBW infants.[68,69] NEC remains a major cause of morbidity and mortality, with extremely low-birth-weight infants having the highest rates of disease.[70–72] When compared with a diet of premature infant formula, preterm infants fed their mother's milk have improved feeding tolerance and a lower incidence of late-onset sepsis and NEC.[5] The use of bovine milk–based fortifiers, while needed to improve nutritional adequacy of PHM, may contribute to the onset of NEC.

A reduction in NEC, both medical and surgical, was reported more than 20 years ago among infants who received only human milk when compared with infants less than 1850 g birth weight who received all bovine milk–based formula.[73] Those infants who received a mixture of formula and human milk had an intermediate level of protection. This study preceded the use of powdered fortifiers for PHM. A contemporary re-evaluation of this older study was done recently, including fortifiers as part of the nutritional management of infants with birth weight of 500 to 1250 g.[7] Infants whose mothers intended to provide their own milk were randomized to an all-human milk regimen (own mother's milk, DHM supplement, all human milk fortifier) or human milk–bovine regimen (human milk, bovine formula/fortifier supplement). Within the all-human milk group, infants were fortified at 40 mL/k/d or 100 mL/k/d. The infants receiving an exclusively human milk-based diet had significantly lower rates of NEC and surgical NEC when compared with those that also received bovine milk–based products: 4.5% and 7% in the all human milk groups, respectively, compared with 16% in the human milk–bovine group. The rate of surgical NEC in infants receiving only human milk was 1.5% compared with 12% in those receiving the human milk–bovine diet.

The background rates of NEC in the study centers were higher than that seen in benchmark data from large networks and reports from many NICUs.[68,69] The study was originally powered to evaluate days of total parenteral nutrition as a surrogate for improved tolerance with exclusive human milk. However, statistical significance was reached because of the magnitude of the NEC observed in those units. The data from this study suggested that the number needed to treat (NNT) with an all-human feeding protocol to prevent 1 case of NEC was 10, and the NNT to prevent 1 case of surgical NEC or death was 8. The authors concluded that no other intervention has had such a marked effect on the incidence of NEC.[7]

It is impossible to determine whether the lower rate of NEC seen in the human milk arm was due to the benefit of the human milk fortifier or to the benefit of giving human milk as opposed to bovine formula milk. Another small randomized study feeding an exclusively human milk–based diet with donor milk and the human fortifier compared with preterm bovine milk formula showed a reduction in days of total parenteral nutrition and a lower rate of surgical NEC in the exclusive human milk diet.[74] The groups included 24 (bovine formula) and 29 (all human milk) infants with mean birth weights of approximately 1000 g. Surgical NEC in the bovine formula group was statistically significantly higher (17%) compared with none in the all human milk group. The authors suggest that this study adds more evidence that all-human milk diets are important for mitigating the morbidity and mortality of NEC.

In a recent letter to the editor in *Breastfeeding Medicine*, Embleton and colleagues[75] suggested that an unequivocal case for the use of the all human milk fortifier has not been determined. They recommended that a definitive and appropriately powered trial should be done to test these results further, using more common estimates of NEC incidence.

The evidence that human milk provides VLBW infants with benefits related to immunity, tolerance, and neurodevelopment is indisputable. Providing milk for her infant is invaluable for the mother and her infant. Benefits persist through the NICU period and beyond. However, human milk alone is nutritionally inadequate for the rapid growth of the VLBW infant during a critical window for brain development. In 2013, there are products and technological devices that can be used to assist the clinician in meeting the needs of these vulnerable infants.

REFERENCES

1. American Academy of Pediatrics Section on Breastfeeding. Breastfeeding and the use of human milk. Pediatrics 2012;129(3):e827–41.
2. Furman L, Taylor G, Minich N, et al. The effect of maternal milk on neonatal morbidity of very low-birth-weight infants. Arch Pediatr Adolesc Med 2003; 157(1):66–71.
3. Patel AL, Johnson TJ, Engstrom JL, et al. Impact of early human milk on sepsis and health-care costs in very low birth weight infants. J Perinatol 2013;33:514–9.
4. Schanler RJ. The use of human milk for premature infants. Pediatr Clin North Am 2001;48(1):207–19.
5. Schanler RJ, Shulman RJ, Lau C. Feeding strategies for premature infants: beneficial outcomes of feeding fortified human milk versus preterm formula. Pediatrics 1999;103(6 Pt 1):1150–7.
6. Sisk PM, Lovelady CA, Dillard RG, et al. Early human milk feeding is associated with a lower risk of necrotizing enterocolitis in very low birth weight infants. J Perinatol 2007;27(7):428–33.
7. Sullivan S, Schanler RJ, Kim JH, et al. An exclusively human milk-based diet is associated with a lower rate of necrotizing enterocolitis than a diet of human milk and bovine milk-based products. J Pediatr 2010;156(4):562–7.e1.

8. Vohr BR, Poindexter BB, Dusick AM, et al. Persistent beneficial effects of breast milk ingested in the neonatal intensive care unit on outcomes of extremely low birth weight infants at 30 months of age. Pediatrics 2007;120(4):e953–9.

9. Schanler R. Evaluation of the evidence to support current recommendations to meet the needs of premature infants: the role of human milk. Am J Clin Nutr 2007;85(2):625S–8S.

10. Bier JA, Oliver T, Ferguson AE, et al. Human milk improves cognitive and motor development of premature infants during infancy. J Hum Lact 2002;18(4):361–7.

11. Blaymore Bier JA, Oliver T, Ferguson A, et al. Human milk reduces outpatient upper respiratory symptoms in premature infants during their first year of life. J Perinatol 2002;22:354–9.

12. Lucas A, Morley R, Cole TJ. Randomised trial of early diet in preterm babies and later intelligence quotient. BMJ 1998;317(7171):1481–7.

13. Morales Y, Schanler RJ. Human milk and clinical outcomes in VLBW infants: how compelling is the evidence of benefit? Semin Perinatol 2007;31(2):83–8.

14. Meinzen-Derr J, Poindexter B, Wrage L, et al. Role of human milk in extremely low birth weight infants' risk of necrotizing enterocolitis or death. J Perinatol 2009;29(1):57–62.

15. Narayanan I, Prakash K, Murthy NS, et al. Randomised controlled trial of effect of raw and holder pasteurised human milk and of formula supplements on incidence of neonatal infection. Lancet 1984;2(8412):1111–3.

16. Lemons JA, Moye L, Hall D, et al. Differences in the composition of preterm and term human milk during early lactation. Pediatr Res 1982;16(2):113–7.

17. Michaelsen KF, Skafte L, Badsberg JH, et al. Variation in macronutrients in human bank milk: influencing factors and implications for human milk banking. J Pediatr Gastroenterol Nutr 1990;11(2):229–39.

18. Wojcik KY, Rechtman DJ, Lee ML, et al. Macronutrient analysis of a nationwide sample of donor breast milk. J Am Diet Assoc 2009;109:137–40.

19. Ziegler EE. Breast-milk fortification. Acta Paediatr 2001;90(7):720–3.

20. Allen JC, Keller RP, Archer P, et al. Studies in human lactation: milk composition and daily secretion rates of macronutrients in the first year of lactation. Am J Clin Nutr 1991;54(1):69–80.

21. Daly SE, Di Rosso A, Owens RA, et al. Degree of breast emptying explains changes in the fat content, but not fatty acid composition, of human milk. Exp Physiol 1993;78(6):741–55.

22. Mitoulas LR, Kent JC, Cox DB, et al. Variation in fat, lactose and protein in human milk over 24 h and throughout the first year of lactation. Br J Nutr 2002; 88(1):29–37.

23. Bhatia J. Human milk and the premature infant. J Perinatol 2007;27:S71–4.

24. Polberger S. New approaches to optimizing early diets. Nestle Nutr Workshop Ser Pediatr Program 2009;63:195–204 [discussion: 204–8, 259–68].

25. Weber A, Loui A, Jochum F, et al. Breast milk from mothers of very low birth-weight infants: variability in fat and protein content. Acta Paediatr 2001;90(7): 772–5.

26. Bertino E, Coppa GV, Giuliani F, et al. Effects of Holder pasteurization on human milk oligosaccharides. Int J Immunopathol Pharmacol 2008;21(2):381–5.

27. Ewaschuk JB, Unger S, O'Connor DL, et al. Effect of pasteurization on selected immune components of donated human breast milk. J Perinatol 2011;31(9):593–8.

28. McPherson RJ, Wagner CL. The effect of pasteurization on transforming growth factor alpha and transforming growth factor beta 2 concentrations in human milk. Adv Exp Med Biol 2001;501:559–66.

29. Untalan PB, Keeney SE, Palkowetz KH, et al. Heat susceptibility of interleukin-10 and other cytokines in donor human milk. Breastfeed Med 2009;4(3):137–44.
30. Silvestre D, Ruiz P, Martinez-Costa C, et al. Effect of pasteurization on the bactericidal capacity of human milk. J Hum Lact 2008;24(4):371–6.
31. Vieira AA, Soares FV, Pimenta HP, et al. Analysis of the influence of pasteurization, freezing/thawing, and offer processes on human milk's macronutrient concentrations. Early Hum Dev 2011;87(8):577–80.
32. Ehrenkranz RA, Dusick AM, Vohr BR, et al. Growth in the neonatal intensive care unit influences neurodevelopmental and growth outcomes of extremely low birth weight infants. Pediatrics 2006;117(4):1253–61.
33. Weisglas-Kuperus N, Hille ET, Duivenvoorden HJ, et al. Intelligence of very preterm or very low birthweight infants in young adulthood. Arch Dis Child Fetal Neonatal Ed 2009;94(3):F196–200.
34. Carlson SJ, Ziegler EE. Nutrient intakes and growth of very low birth weight infants. J Perinatol 1998;18(4):252–8.
35. Embleton NE, Pang N, Cooke RJ. Postnatal malnutrition and growth retardation: an inevitable consequence of current recommendations in preterm infants? Pediatrics 2001;107(2):270–3.
36. Latal-Hajnal B, von Siebenthal K, Kovari H, et al. Postnatal growth in VLBW infants: significant association with neurodevelopmental outcome. J Pediatr 2003;143(2):163–70.
37. Kiechl-Kohlendorfer U, Fink FM, Steichen-Gersdorf E. Transient symptomatic zinc deficiency in a breast-fed preterm infant. Pediatr Dermatol 2007;24(5):536–40.
38. Obladen M, Loui A, Kampmann W, et al. Zinc deficiency in rapidly growing preterm infants. Acta Paediatr 1998;87(6):685–91.
39. Arslanoglu S, Moro GE, Ziegler EE, The Wapm Working Group On Nutrition. Optimization of human milk fortification for preterm infants: new concepts and recommendations. J Perinat Med 2010;38(3):233–8.
40. Rigo J. Protein, amino acid and other nitrogen compounds. In: Tsang RC, Uauy R, Koletzko B, et al, editors. Nutrition of the preterm infant: scientific basis and practical guidelines. 2nd edition. Cincinnati (OH): Digital Educational Publishing, Inc; 2005. p. 45.
41. Arslanoglu S, Moro GE, Ziegler EE. Preterm infants fed fortified human milk receive less protein than they need. J Perinatol 2009;29(7):489–92.
42. de Halleux V, Rigo J. Variability in human milk composition: benefit of individualized fortification in very low birth weight infants. Am J Clin Nutr 2013;98(2):529S–35S.
43. Senterre T, Rigo J. Optimizing early nutritional support based on recent recommendations in VLBW infants and postnatal growth restriction. J Pediatr Gastroenterol Nutr 2011;53(5):536–42.
44. Baker RD. Infant formula safety. Pediatrics 2002;110(4):833–5.
45. Steele C, Kinzler S. Microbiology and infection control. In: Robbins ST, Meyers R, editors. Infant feedings: guidelines for preparation of human milk and formula in health care facilities. 2nd edition. Chicago: Diana Faulhaber; 2011. p. 108–21.
46. Moya F, Sisk PM, Walsh KR, et al. A new liquid human milk fortifier and linear growth in preterm infants. Pediatrics 2012;130(4):e928–35.
47. Erickson T, Gill G, Chan GM. The effects of acidification on human milk's cellular and nutritional content. J Perinatol 2013;33(5):371–3.
48. Lonnerdal B. Personalizing nutrient intakes of formula-fed infants: breast milk as a model. Nestle Nutr Workshop Ser Pediatr Program 2008;62:189–98 [discussion: 198–203].

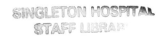
SINGLETON HOSPITAL
STAFF LIBRARY

49. Kuschel CA, Harding JE. Multicomponent fortified human milk for promoting growth in preterm infants. Cochrane Database Syst Rev 2004;(1):CD000343.
50. Olsen IE, Richardson DK, Schmid CH, et al. Intersite differences in weight growth velocity of extremely premature infants. Pediatrics 2002;110(6):1125–32.
51. Pieltain C, De Curtis M, Gerard P, et al. Weight gain composition in preterm infants with dual energy X-ray absorptiometry. Pediatr Res 2001;49(1):120–4.
52. Henriksen C, Westerberg AC, Ronnestad A, et al. Growth and nutrient intake among very-low-birth-weight infants fed fortified human milk during hospitalisation. Br J Nutr 2009;102(8):1179–86.
53. Radmacher PG, Lewis SL, Adamkin D. Individualizing fortification of human milk using real time human milk analysis. J Neonatal Perinatal Med 2013;6:319–23.
54. Arslanoglu S, Moro GE, Ziegler EE. Adjustable fortification of human milk fed to preterm infants: does it make a difference? J Perinatol 2006;26(10):614–21.
55. Hay WW Jr. Optimizing protein intake in preterm infants. J Perinatol 2009;29(7):465–6.
56. Radmacher PG, Sparks B, Lewis SL, et al. Real time human milk analysis contributes to more comprehensive nutritional management. J Investig Med 2013;61(2):208A.
57. Rochow N, Fusch G, Choi A, et al. Target fortification of breast milk with fat, protein and carbohydrates for preterm infants. J Pediatr 2013;163:1001–7.
58. Polberger S, Raiha NC, Juvonen P, et al. Individualized protein fortification of human milk for preterm infants: comparison of ultrafiltrated human milk protein and a bovine whey fortifier. J Pediatr Gastroenterol Nutr 1999;29(3):332–8.
59. O'Neill EF, Radmacher PG, Sparks B, et al. Creamatocrit analysis of human milk overestimates fat and energy content when compared to a human milk analyzer using mid-infrared spectroscopy. J Pediatr Gastroenterol Nutr 2013;56(5):569–73.
60. Sauer CW, Kim JH. Human milk macronutrient analysis using point-of-care near-infrared spectrophotometry. J Perinatol 2011;31(5):339–43.
61. Agostoni C, Buonocore G, Carnielli VP, et al. Enteral nutrient supply for preterm infants: commentary from the European Society of Paediatric Gastroenterology, Hepatology and Nutrition Committee on Nutrition. J Pediatr Gastroenterol Nutr 2010;50(1):85–91.
62. AOAC. Official method 972.16. Fat, lactose, protein, and solids in milk. Mid-infrared spectroscopic method. In: Horitz W, editor. Official methods of analysis, vol. 2, 17th edition. Gaithersburg (MD): AOAC International; 2003.
63. Biggs DA, Johnsson G, Sjaunja LO. Analysis of fat, protein, lactose and total solids by infra-red absorption. Monograph on Rapid Indirect Methods for Measurement of the Major Conponents of Milk. Bulletin of the International Dairy Federation 208. Brussels (Belgium): International Dairy Federation; 1987. p. 21–30.
64. Biggs DA, McKenna D. Alternative methods for infrared analysis of fat in milk: interlaboratory study. J Assoc Off Anal Chem 1989;72:724–34.
65. Casadio YS, Williams TM, Lai CT, et al. Evaluation of a mid-infrared analyzer for the determination of the macronutrient composition of human milk. J Hum Lact 2010;26(4):376–83.
66. Sjaunja L-O. Studies on milk analysis of individual cow milk samples. I. Infrared spectrophotometry for analysis of fat, protein and lactose in milk. Acta Agric Scand 1984;34(3):249–59.
67. Corvaglia L, Battistini B, Paoletti V, et al. Near-infrared reflectance analysis to evaluate the nitrogen and fat content of human milk in neonatal intensive care units. Arch Dis Child Fetal Neonatal Ed 2008;93:F372–5.

68. Lin PW, Stoll BJ. Necrotising enterocolitis. Lancet 2006;368(9543):1271–83.
69. Stoll BJ. Epidemiology of necrotizing enterocolitis. Clin Perinatol 1994;21(2): 205–18.
70. Horbar JD, Badger GJ, Carpenter JH, et al. Trends in mortality and morbidity for very low birth weight infants, 1991-1999. Pediatrics 2002;110(1 Pt 1):143–51.
71. Lemons JA, Bauer CR, Oh W, et al. Very low birth weight outcomes of the National Institute of Child health and human development neonatal research network, January 1995 through December 1996. NICHD Neonatal Research Network. Pediatrics 2001;107(1):E1.
72. Peter CS, Feuerhahn M, Bohnhorst B, et al. Necrotising enterocolitis: is there a relationship to specific pathogens? Eur J Pediatr 1999;158(1):67–70.
73. Lucas A, Cole TJ. Breast milk and neonatal necrotising enterocolitis. Lancet 1990;336(8730):1519–23.
74. Cristofalo EA, Schanler R, Blanco C, et al. Randomized trial of exclusive human milk versus preterm formula diets in extremely premature infants. J Pediatr 2013; 163(6):1592–5.
75. Embleton ND, King C, Jarvis C, et al. Effectiveness of human milk-based fortifiers for preventing NEC in preterm infants: case not proven. Breastfeed Med 2013;8(4):421.

Human Breast Milk and the Gastrointestinal Innate Immune System

Brett M. Jakaitis, MD, Patricia W. Denning, MD*

KEYWORDS

- Mucosal innate immune system • Human breast milk • Bioactive factors
- Lactoferrin • Antimicrobial peptides • Commensal bacteria • Intestinal microbiome

KEY POINTS

- Newborns infants are in a susceptible immunologic state after birth, with an immature adaptive immune system, making them reliant on their innate immune system for protection.
- The gastrointestinal innate immune system is comprised of many components. The acidic environment in the stomach and the mucus layer of the small intestine provide an initial barrier. The intestinal epithelial cells create a physical barrier and are involved in signaling to the underlying tissue. The lamina propria is rich in immune cells and contributes greatly to intestinal defense.
- In addition to providing optimal nutrition to infants, human breast milk has an abundance of bioactive factors that act as a part of the innate immune system of the gastrointestinal tract. Some factors have intrinsic properties that act as part of the defense system, whereas others enhance the ability of the gastrointestinal tract to defend the host.

INTRODUCTION

The epithelial layers and mucus secretions of the pulmonary, genitourinary, and gastrointestinal (GI) systems all provide a complex mechanical barrier and an inherent defense against pathogens that constantly threaten the human body. Evidence suggests that these systems do not work independently, but form what is referred to as the mucosal immunologic system, an integrated network of tissue, cells, and signaling molecules.[1] Of the 3 systems, the lining of the GI tract provides the largest interface with the external environment (200–300 m^2). Although it was long believed to exist solely for food digestion and nutrient absorption, it is now known that the responsibilities of the intestinal system are diverse and critical to host defense. This amazing organ has evolved an elaborate defense system to protect the human body from

Division of Neonatology, Department of Pediatrics, Emory University School of Medicine, 2015 Uppergate Drive, 3rd Floor, Atlanta, GA 30322, USA
* Corresponding author.
E-mail address: pllin@emory.edu

Clin Perinatol 41 (2014) 423–435
http://dx.doi.org/10.1016/j.clp.2014.02.011
0095-5108/14/$ – see front matter © 2014 Elsevier Inc. All rights reserved.

continuous threats of numerous disease-causing agents and commensal bacteria present at an impressive number (1×10^{14} CFU).[2] At no time in life is this function more important than shortly after birth. The infant's abrupt introduction to life outside the uterus and exposure to antigens forces the GI tract to adapt quickly and commence its crucial duties. But the neonate's adaptive immune system is naive, and the developmental immunologic immaturity leaves the newborn in a state of vulnerability and at increased risk for serious infection. Components of the intestinal innate immune system do not rely on memory and can act with a preformed, nonspecific response.

Feeding exclusively with human milk is recommended for the first 6 months of life[3] and provides unique components and nutrients, leading to optimal nutrition, growth, and development of the newborn infant.[4] The benefits of human breast milk and its association with healthier babies have been intermittently noted over the past few thousand years.[5] In 1934, Grulee and colleagues[6] showed that formula-fed infants had higher morbidity and mortality when compared with breastfed infants. More recently, breast milk has been associated with a decreased incidence of necrotizing enterocolitis (NEC),[7] gastroenteritis,[8] severe respiratory illness,[9] otitis media,[10–14] and urinary tract infections.[15] The unique and dynamic composition of human milk not only supplies optimal nutrients but also contributes an abundance of bioactive factors,[16] which support and enhance the deficient immunologic system of the newborn.

In this article, selected factors in breast milk and how they either act alone to provide innate protection or augment GI innate immune function are reviewed. First, a broad and brief overview of innate immunity within the intestinal system is provided. Then, individual constituents present in human breast milk and the variety of mechanisms by which they exert their effects and afford protection to the newborn infant are discussed.

THE INNATE IMMUNE SYSTEM OF THE GI TRACT

The complex immune system of the intestine can be divided into 2 broad categories: innate and adaptive immunity. Although the innate arm, as its name implies, is present from birth and capable of immediate protection at the local level, the adaptive immune system of the gut is initially naive and needs time to generate an appropriate response and memory. Although much of our focus is on the components of innate immunity in the gut, it is important to remember that this system does not work in isolation. The information it gathers communicates with the adaptive immune system, allowing the 2 to work in concert to provide optimal protection for the host. The innate defense system of the intestine can be broken down into 3 main components: the secreted mucus layer within the gut lumen, a single intestinal epithelial cell (IEC) layer, and the underlying lamina propria.

Mucus Layer

Large, highly glycosylated proteins called mucins are secreted by specialized goblet cells,[17,18] also known as mucin-secreting cells, and are the primary component of mucus. The mucus layer, which is present throughout the GI tract, provides protection, lubrication, and compartmentalization, minimizing contact between the epithelium and commensal bacteria. Mucins secreted by salivary glands coat food and assist with esophageal transit.[19] The mucus layer in the stomach plays a role in protecting the epithelium from the harsh acidic environment.[19] The gel-forming mucin, MUC2, is the most predominant mucin in both the small and large intestine.[20] There is 1 unattached layer of mucin in the small intestine, which acts as a physical and chemical barrier, preventing pathogenic bacteria from contacting the intestinal epithelia.[21] The colon has 2 distinct mucus layers, with the outer layer containing many bacteria and the inner layer being resistant to bacterial penetration.[22] Attached to the apical side of enterocytes in the small intestine is a separate, thin layer of mucus, made up of transmembrane mucins. This layer is commonly referred to as the glycocalyx; it affords protection to the IECs by means of a physical barrier and plays a role in cellular signaling.[23] An abnormal mucus layer may lead to both acute and chronic intestinal diseases and has been shown to be associated with colitis in a murine model.[24]

Antimicrobial peptides (AMPs), a critical element in the chemical response of the innate immune system, are released into the mucus layer of the intestine. These small peptides (20–40 amino acids long) are secreted by the Paneth cell, a pyramidal columnar exocrine cell located at the base of the crypts of Lieberkühn, and can respond to a threat within a matter of hours. The continual release of AMPs by Paneth cells maintains the relatively sterile environment of the intestinal crypt, where the intestinal epithelial stem cells reside. When stimulated by inflammatory mediators, AMPs are also secreted into the lumen to help with mucosal defense.[23] They have microbicidal activity against a wide range of pathogens, including many gram-negative and gram-positive bacteria, fungi, protozoa, and viruses.[18] Paneth cell dysfunction has been shown to lead to decreased clearance of pathogenic *Escherichia coli*.[25] Several AMPs are present in the neonate's intestine. Some of the most important and abundant are α-defensin, β-defensin, lysozyme, and LL-37 (a member of the cathelicidin family).

IECs

The intestinal epithelial layer is made up of 4 different types of cells: absorptive enterocytes, hormone-secreting enteroendocrine cells, mucus-secreting goblet cells, and antimicrobial-secreting Paneth cells. These cells mature from a common pluripotent stem cell located in the base of the crypts. This single layer of highly polarized IECs sits below the mucus layer, creating a physical barrier that is anchored by junctional proteins. They are also responsible for sampling intraluminal contents, which instigates transcellular signaling and transcription of genes, resulting in a defense response via the release of cytokines and chemokines and subsequent attraction of leukocytes. This function is mediated by multiple pattern recognition receptors (PRRs), critical for the identification of foreign elements such as peptidoglycan, lipoproteins, viral DNA, and commensal microflora. The remarkable ability of these receptors to distinguish between harmful and helpful bacteria with subsequent appropriate signaling is critical to intestinal homeostasis.[26] Toll-like receptors (TLRs) are the predominant type of PRR found on the apical side of IECs. Another group of PRRs that cooperate with TLRs are the intracellular NOD-like receptors (NLRs). NOD1 is expressed by IECs, and NOD2 is found in monocytes, dendritic cells, and Paneth cells.[23]

Tight junctions (TJs) regulate paracellular permeability and maintain separation of tissue compartments by sealing the intercellular space[27,28] and are an essential component of the epithelial barrier. A breakdown in the functioning of TJs and, subsequently, the intestinal immune barrier has been implicated in the pathogenesis of idiopathic inflammatory bowel disease,[29,30] infectious enteritis, and NEC.[31] Three types of proteins make up TJs: occludins, claudins, and junctional adhesion molecules. Although not much is known about the occludin proteins, it is known that the family of claudin proteins control the size, strength, and specificity of the ions that can pass through the epithelium.[23] In addition to TJs, adherens junctions are present on the lateral side of the epithelial cells and facilitate intercellular signaling.

Lamina Propria

A comprehensive review of the innate and adaptive immune functions occurring within the lamina propria is beyond the scope of this article. Further, the gut-associated lymphoid tissue include Peyer patches, isolated lymphoid follicles, and M cells, which are not discussed in this review. Intraepithelial T-cell lymphocytes have also recently been recognized as an important innate immune cell, which is critical for host-microbial homeostasis and protects the gut from injury.[32] The lamina propria contains many innate immune cells; the functions of these cells are being elucidated in ongoing animal and human studies. Among these cells are macrophages and dendritic cells; their roles include antigen uptake and transport, induction of T-cell differentiation, stimulation of immunoglobulin production (IgA), and tissue repair.[33] Macrophages and dendritic cells are also important for maintaining tolerance to the commensal microbiota.[33] In addition to different populations of T-cell and B-cell lymphocytes present in the lamina propria, innate lymphoid cell populations have recently been described, including natural killer cells, which are purported to play important roles in producing proinflammatory and regulatory cytokines.[34]

There certainly are other components of the innate immune system, which are not discussed here but are important. One simple example is the acidic and bacteriocidal environment of the stomach, which not only aids in digestion but also decreases the number of viable pathogens reaching the distal intestine. The disruption of this milieu can lead to disease. Multiple studies have revealed an association between the use of histamine 2 blockers, which inhibit gastric acid secretion, and both NEC and late-onset sepsis.[35–38]

INNATE IMMUNITY AND HUMAN BREAST MILK

Human infants are born with certain developmental immune deficiencies.[39] Phagocyte function and responses are immature and inadequate. Antibody production is limited and delayed, and serum IgA levels are far lower than adult levels. Both the classic and alternative pathways of the complement cascade have decreased performance. In addition to nutritive components, the ingestion of human breast milk delivers numerous antipathogenic and antiinflammatory bioactive factors[40] that provide passive protection to the neonate and stimulate maturation of host intestinal defenses. This factor is particularly relevant for premature infants, whose immune defenses are more immature than term neonates. The milk of mothers who give birth prematurely contains higher amounts of phagocytes and secretory immunoglobulin A (sIgA).[41–43] Breast milk is capable of directly modulating the development of the immune system,[44] as breastfed infants have been shown to have a reduced incidence of allergic disease[45] and autoimmune diseases such as Crohn disease[46] and insulin-dependent diabetes mellitus.[47] These collective properties make breast milk the gold standard for providing protective nutrients to the newborn.[48]

The Intestinal Microbial Environment

Colonization of the infant gut with more than 400 species of commensal bacteria lays the foundation for a healthy microbiome, which contributes to immune homeostasis, setting up a symbiotic relationship between colonizing bacteria and the underlying epithelial cells and lamina propria.[49,50] Barrier function, mucin and IgA secretion, inflammation, and homeostatic processes such as proliferation and apoptosis are influenced by these helpful bacteria.[51–56] Their effects on the intestinal immune system are believed to be largely mediated through TLRs present on IECs, which are able to distinguish between commensal bacteria and harmful pathogens.[57] Normal colonization begins at the time of birth with a vaginal delivery, when the infant is exposed to maternal vaginal and colonic bacteria. This process is followed by an exclusive diet of human milk, which contains factors that promote the growth of commensal bacteria. Distinct differences have been shown in the intestinal flora of breastfed and bottle-fed infants.[58]

Oligosaccharides are nondigestable sugars found in breast milk and are believed to be responsible for promoting the growth of protective bacteria in the colon. They make up approximately 1% of the milk and 10% of the caloric content,[59] although the amount present varies diurnally and with duration of lactation and the infant's gestational age.[60] The presence of a nonnutritional substance at such high concentrations led to the hypothesis that glycans, including oligosaccharides, play a role in protection against disease. Because they are indigestible, oligosaccharides pass through the small intestine and enter the colon. Here, they produce short-chain fatty acids through fermentation, creating a favorable environment for the growth of probiotic bacterial species such as bifidobacteria and lactobacilli. This factor leads to a stable ecosystem in the intestine and augmentation of intestinal host defenses. The stimulation of sIgA-producing plasma cells in the intestine by these commensal bacteria is 1 such example of this symbiotic relationship.[61] Furthermore, glycans can inhibit binding of pathogens to the intestinal cell wall by acting as ligands, attaching to various bacteria, toxins, and viruses.[62]

sIgA

In the human adult, large amounts of sIgA are produced daily by plasma cells in the gut and transported into the intestinal lumen. This abundant antibody coats both harmful and commensal microorganisms, preventing colonization and penetration of the mucosal barrier, and it may even be able to inactivate certain viruses.[63] In the full-term newborn gut, plasma cells responsible for producing sIgA are absent for about 10 days after birth, and it takes up to 30 days postpartum for the neonatal intestine to produce levels of sIgA that are sufficient for protection.[64] To compensate for this deficiency, maternal milk contains large amounts of sIgA, which accounts for 90% of total immunoglobulins in milk. More than 50 years ago, it was discovered that there was up to 12 g/L of sIgA in human colostrum and 1 g/L in mature milk.[65] When secreted by the infant's gut, sIgA can be considered a part of the innate immune system, but when sIgA is ingested in mother's milk, it works through a unique system of immunity whereby the infant acquires protection from enteric pathogens to which the mother is exposed. First, within the mother's intestine, a novel enteric pathogen is presented to the dendritic cell. Next, activated T lymphocytes stimulate B lymphocytes, inducing the production of IgA by plasma cells at the basolateral side of the mammary epithelial cell. IgA is then transported across the epithelial cell attached to the polyimmunoglobulin receptor. On the apical side, the complex is cleaved, and dimeric sIgA is secreted into the milk, conferring immunity to the nursing infant.[66]

Selected Bioactive Proteins in Breast Milk with Antipathogenic Activity

Lactoferrin

This multifunctional, iron-binding glycoprotein possesses many anti-infective properties that act as part of the innate immune system and is present in mature human breast milk at concentrations of 1 to 3 g/L and in colostrum at 7 g/L.[67] It also occurs naturally in most exocrine fluids such as tears, saliva, bile, and pancreatic secretions. A recent study performed in very low birth weight infants showed that administration of bovine lactoferrin (LF), which is nearly homologous with human LF, either alone or in combination with *LGG*, can reduce the incidence of late-onset sepsis caused by bacteria and invasive fungal infections.[68,69] Antiviral properties have also been shown against a wide range of viruses, including human immunodeficiency virus, cytomegalovirus, herpes simplex virus, hepatitis B and C, adenovirus, and rotavirus.[70]

Many modes of action have been discovered by which LF acts to provide protection to the neonate, including its high affinity for iron, which may limit the amount of iron available to bacteria and other microorganisms. When LF is exposed to pepsin in the stomach, a potent antimicrobial agent is produced called lactoferricin, which is capable of killing a wide range of pathogens and, in particular, disrupts the cell membrane of gram-negative bacteria.[71] Another factor contained in breast milk, lysozyme, acts together with LF in the stomach to kill gram-negative bacteria.[72] Intact LF is passed into the small intestine and can bind to multiple receptors, including TLRs and CD14, blocking the adherence of pathogens to the intestinal epithelium.[73] Other beneficial actions of LF in the intestine include initiation of apoptosis in infected IECs,[74] promotion of growth of commensal bacteria,[75] stimulation of proliferation and differentiation of IECs,[76] and a reduction in inflammatory cytokine production through inhibition of nuclear factor κB activation in monocytes.[48,77] LF continues to be at the forefront in the fight against systemic infections and NEC in premature infants. There are multiple ongoing clinical trials studies looking at the effects of either bovine LF or human recombinant LF.

Lysozyme

This antibacterial enzyme is present in breast milk at relatively high concentrations. It can act alone to degrade bacteria by cleaving β,1-4 glycoside linkages in their cells walls.[78] As mentioned earlier, the activity of lysozyme can be increased through its relationship with LF. This expansion of its capabilities is accomplished when LF disrupts the outer membrane of gram-negative bacteria, such as *Salmonella typhimurium* and *E coli*. Lysozyme can then enter the bacteria and destroy it.[72]

Caseins

This family of highly glycosylated proteins makes up about 40% of the protein present in human milk and has immunologic activity in the newborn. β-casein is the predominant casein found in human milk. A synthetic peptide of β-casein has been shown to stimulate the expression of MUC2 genes and increase the numbers of goblet cells and Paneth cells in the small intestine of a rat pup model.[79] As discussed earlier, MUC2 is the most prevalent mucin in the mucus layer of the small intestine and provides protection through multiple mechanisms. κ-Casein is a minor casein subunit in breast milk.[80] It can act as a receptor analogue, preventing the attachment of bacteria to mucosal epithelium[81] and inhibit binding of *Helicobacter pylori* to human gastric mucosa in vitro.[82]

Cytokines and Chemokines Found in Human Milk

The gut of the newborn lacks the ability to respond appropriately to foreign pathogens and, more specifically, the capacity to produce a contained inflammatory response. There is a tendency toward excessive inflammatory signaling, as shown in immature IECs when exposed to inflammatory stimuli such as interleukin 1β (IL-1β), tumor necrosis factor α, and lipopolysaccharide, with an increased release of IL-8,[48,83] a chemokine known to stimulate neutrophil recruitment.[84] Cytokines are responsible for mediating, regulating, and modulating immune responses. Human breast milk contains a significant amount of this diverse group of signaling molecules, which help control the inflammatory response. For example, the antiinflammatory cytokine, IL-10, is present in breast milk[85] and believed to be critical for intestinal homeostasis and protection of the host. IL-10–deficient mice develop chronic enterocolitis,[86] and human infants with defects in the genes encoding IL-10 receptor subunit proteins have severe early-onset colitis.[87] With regard to NEC, IL-10 knockout mice have increased intestinal inflammation and increased apoptosis of IECs when exposed to hypoxia and formula feeding,[88] and the feeding of maternal milk in a rat model led to a reduction in the severity of NEC and increased intestinal IL-10.[89] Claud and colleagues[83] found that IL-10 and transforming growth factor β (TGF-β) both decreased IL-8 secretion by fetal human enterocytes in vitro.

The TGF-β family of immunoregulatory cytokines have been shown to be involved in wound healing, the inhibition of inflammation by decreasing the production of proinflammatory cytokines, and the regulation of lymphocytes, natural killer cells, dendritic cells, macrophages, and granulocytes.[90] Neonates have decreased expression of TGF-β,[91] but maternal milk supplies sufficient levels of the much-needed cytokine.[92] Exogenous supplementation can have a significant impact on the developing mucosal immune system, through its effects on oral tolerance and regulatory T cells. Infants breastfed by mothers with increased levels of TGF-β in breast milk have a decreased risk of wheezing and atopic dermatitis in childhood.[93,94] In direct relation to the innate immune system, TGF-β can also initiate local production of IgA in the gut, providing additional protection.[95]

Development and Repair of the GI Epithelium

With exposure to multiple factors in amniotic fluid and human breast milk, growth and differentiation of the intestinal epithelium peak shortly after birth. Epidermal growth factor (EGF) is a peptide that augments IEC proliferation and differentiation[96] and is secreted by multiple cells throughout the GI system into the intestinal lumen. EGF is supplied by amniotic fluid throughout pregnancy, whereas the infant in the postnatal period relies on the significant concentrations of EGF found in human milk and colostrum. Milk from mothers who have delivered an extremely premature infant contains 50% to 80% more EGF when compared with milk from mothers with full-term infants,[97] leading to speculation that EGF may be one of the reasons why human milk is protective against NEC.[98] Enteral administration of EGF resulted in a 50% reduction of NEC in a rat model.[99] More specifically, EGF has been associated with increased goblet cell density and MUC2 production in the ileum, and normalization in the expression of the intestinal epithelial TJ proteins, occluding and claudin, resulting in improved intestinal barrier function.[98,100] Another protein found in human milk that is capable of contributing to the development of the epithelium is LF. In addition to its antibacterial activity discussed earlier, experiments in human intestinal cell lines have shown that LF, which peaks in colostrum, induces cell proliferation at high concentrations and cell differentiation at low concentrations.[76]

Other Active Components in Breast Milk

Leukocytes

During early lactation, human milk contains large amounts of macrophages (up to 80% of total cells present), and an infant may consume up to 10^{10} maternal leukocytes per day.[16] Breast milk phagocytes, which are believed to be derived from maternal peripheral blood monocytes, possess unique functional features. One study showed that after phagocytosis of breast milk components, the phagocytes were capable of spontaneously producing granulocyte-macrophage colony-stimulating factor and differentiating into dendritic cells.[101] There is speculation that these cells possess many more functions that we do not yet know about.

Table 1
Selected components present in human breast milk that act as part of the GI innate immune system

Component in Breast Milk	Action	Reference
Oligosaccharides (or prebiotics)	Promote growth of commensal bacteria Directly bind pathogenic bacteria and viruses	62
Secretory IgA	Coats harmful and commensal bacteria, preventing penetration of the epithelial barrier	63
LF	Binds iron within gut and limits its availability to microorganisms Produces lactoferricin when exposed to pepsin Binds receptors, interfering with pathogen binding to the epithelial barrier Stimulation of proliferation and differentiation of IECs Reduces inflammatory cytokine production Induces IEC proliferation and differentiation	48,71,73,76,77
Lysozyme	Degrades bacterial cell walls	78
Casein proteins	Increase numbers of goblet cells, Paneth cells, and expression of MUC2 genes Can act as receptor analogues	79,81
IL-10	Attenuates inflammation in the gut	83
TGF-β	Stimulates local production of sIgA in the gut Regulation of multiple types of immune cells	95
EGF	Increases goblet cell density and MUC2 production in ileum Normalizes expression of TJ proteins	98,100
Free fatty acids and monoglycerides	Antiviral, antibacterial, and antiprotozoal activity in stomach	39,66,102

Triglycerides

The fat or triglyceride found in human milk is a key constituent for infant nutrition and growth. It also has an additional function. When the triglyceride enters the stomach, it is digested by lingual and gastric lipases. This process releases free fatty acids and monoglycerides. These products act as a part of the innate immune system in the stomach and provide immediate protection to the newborn infant through their lytic effect on various viruses and some antibacterial and even antiprotozoal activity, specifically against *Giardia* (**Table 1**).[39,66,102]

SUMMARY

The neonatal intestine faces many changes, including adaptation from a sterile intrauterine environment to one in which a diverse microbial population outnumbers human cells 10 to 1. To maintain homeostasis, it must protect the host from potential noxious and infectious stimuli and tolerate the diverse commensal microbes that colonize the entire gut. Furthermore, the gut must also perform important digestive and absorptive functions. Human breast milk contains many components that aid neonatal gut function and development. Understanding both neonatal gut immunity and how breast milk components influence its development and function are areas of active investigation. Future studies in this field are needed to develop targeted strategies to prevent and treat neonatal gut injury and infection, particularly in extremely low birth weight and premature infants.

REFERENCES

1. Gill N, Wlodarska M, Finlay BB. The future of mucosal immunology: studying an integrated system-wide organ. Nat Immunol 2010;11(7):558–60.
2. Berg RD. The indigenous gastrointestinal microflora. Trends Microbiol 1996; 4(11):430–5.
3. Section on Breastfeeding. Breastfeeding and the use of human milk. Pediatrics 2012;129(3):e827–41.
4. Lonnerdal B. Breast milk: a truly functional food. Nutrition 2000;16(7–8):509–11.
5. Newburg DS. Innate immunity and human milk. J Nutr 2005;135(5):1308–12.
6. Grulee CG, Sanford HN, Herron PH. Breast and artificial feeding. J Am Med Assoc 1934;103:735–8.
7. Lucas A, Cole TJ. Breast milk and neonatal necrotising enterocolitis. Lancet 1990;336(8730):1519–23.
8. Strand TA, Sharma PR, Gjessing HK, et al. Risk factors for extended duration of acute diarrhea in young children. PLoS One 2012;7(5):e36436.
9. Bachrach VR, Schwarz E, Bachrach LR. Breastfeeding and the risk of hospitalization for respiratory disease in infancy: a meta-analysis. Arch Pediatr Adolesc Med 2003;157(3):237–43.
10. Duncan B, Ey J, Holberg CJ, et al. Exclusive breast-feeding for at least 4 months protects against otitis media. Pediatrics 1993;91(5):867–72.
11. Dewey KG, Heinig MJ, Nommsen-Rivers LA. Differences in morbidity between breast-fed and formula-fed infants. J Pediatr 1995;126(5 Pt 1):696–702.
12. Beaudry M, Dufour R, Marcoux S. Relation between infant feeding and infections during the first six months of life. J Pediatr 1995;126(2):191–7.
13. Scariati PD, Grummer-Strawn LM, Fein SB. A longitudinal analysis of infant morbidity and the extent of breastfeeding in the United States. Pediatrics 1997;99(6):E5.
14. Duffy LC, Faden H, Wasielewski R, et al. Exclusive breastfeeding protects against bacterial colonization and day care exposure to otitis media. Pediatrics 1997;100(4):E7.
15. Marild S, Hansson S, Jodal U, et al. Protective effect of breastfeeding against urinary tract infection. Acta Paediatr 2004;93(2):164–8.
16. Ballard O, Morrow AL. Human milk composition: nutrients and bioactive factors. Pediatr Clin North Am 2013;60(1):49–74.
17. Laboisse C, Jarry A, Branka JE, et al. Regulation of mucin exocytosis from intestinal goblet cells. Biochem Soc Trans 1995;23(4):810–3.
18. Lievin-Le Moal V, Servin AL. The front line of enteric host defense against unwelcome intrusion of harmful microorganisms: mucins, antimicrobial peptides, and microbiota. Clin Microbiol Rev 2006;19(2):315–37.
19. Johansson ME, Sjovall H, Hansson GC. The gastrointestinal mucus system in health and disease. Nat Rev Gastroenterol Hepatol 2013;10(6):352–61.
20. Johansson ME, Ambort D, Pelaseyed T, et al. Composition and functional role of the mucus layers in the intestine. Cell Mol Life Sci 2011;68(22):3635–41.
21. Johansson ME, Larsson JM, Hansson GC. The two mucus layers of colon are organized by the MUC2 mucin, whereas the outer layer is a legislator of host-microbial interactions. Proc Natl Acad Sci U S A 2011;108(Suppl 1): 4659–65.
22. Johansson ME, Phillipson M, Petersson J, et al. The inner of the two Muc2 mucin-dependent mucus layers in colon is devoid of bacteria. Proc Natl Acad Sci U S A 2008;105(39):15064–9.

23. McElroy SJ, Weitkamp JH. Innate immunity in the small intestine of the preterm infant. Neoreviews 2011;12(9):e517–26.

24. Heazlewood CK, Cook MC, Eri R, et al. Aberrant mucin assembly in mice causes endoplasmic reticulum stress and spontaneous inflammation resembling ulcerative colitis. PLoS Med 2008;5(3):e54.

25. Sherman MP, Bennett SH, Hwang FF, et al. Paneth cells and antibacterial host defense in neonatal small intestine. Infect Immun 2005;73(9):6143–6.

26. Rakoff-Nahoum S, Paglino J, Eslami-Varzaneh F, et al. Recognition of commensal microflora by toll-like receptors is required for intestinal homeostasis. Cell 2004;118(2):229–41.

27. Anderson JM, Van Itallie CM. Tight junctions. Curr Biol 2008;18(20):R941–3.

28. Balda MS, Fallon MB, Van Itallie CM, et al. Structure, regulation, and pathophysiology of tight junctions in the gastrointestinal tract. Yale J Biol Med 1992;65(6): 725–35 [discussion: 737–40].

29. Clayburgh DR, Shen L, Turner JR. A porous defense: the leaky epithelial barrier in intestinal disease. Lab Invest 2004;84(3):282–91.

30. Sartor RB. Microbial influences in inflammatory bowel diseases. Gastroenterology 2008;134(2):577–94.

31. Henry MC, Moss RL. Neonatal necrotizing enterocolitis. Semin Pediatr Surg 2008;17(2):98–109.

32. Ismail AS, Behrendt CL, Hooper LV. Reciprocal interactions between commensal bacteria and gamma delta intraepithelial lymphocytes during mucosal injury. J Immunol 2009;182(5):3047–54.

33. Varol C, Zigmond E, Jung S. Securing the immune tightrope: mononuclear phagocytes in the intestinal lamina propria. Nat Rev Immunol 2010;10(6): 415–26.

34. Spits H, Di Santo JP. The expanding family of innate lymphoid cells: regulators and effectors of immunity and tissue remodeling. Nat Immunol 2011;12(1):21–7.

35. More K, Athalye-Jape G, Rao S, et al. Association of inhibitors of gastric acid secretion and higher incidence of necrotizing enterocolitis in preterm very low-birth-weight infants. Am J Perinatol 2013;30(10):849–56.

36. Terrin G, Passariello A, De Curtis M, et al. Ranitidine is associated with infections, necrotizing enterocolitis, and fatal outcome in newborns. Pediatrics 2012;129(1):e40–5.

37. Bianconi S, Gudavalli M, Sutija VG, et al. Ranitidine and late-onset sepsis in the neonatal intensive care unit. J Perinat Med 2007;35(2):147–50.

38. Graham PL 3rd, Begg MD, Larson E, et al. Risk factors for late onset gram-negative sepsis in low birth weight infants hospitalized in the neonatal intensive care unit. Pediatr Infect Dis J 2006;25(2):113–7.

39. Lawrence RM, Pane CA. Human breast milk: current concepts of immunology and infectious diseases. Curr Probl Pediatr Adolesc Health Care 2007;37(1): 7–36.

40. Goldman AS. The immune system of human milk: antimicrobial, antiinflammatory and immunomodulating properties. Pediatr Infect Dis J 1993;12(8):664–71.

41. Gross SJ, Buckley RH, Wakil SS, et al. Elevated IgA concentration in milk produced by mothers delivered of preterm infants. J Pediatr 1981;99(3):389–93.

42. Schlesinger L, Munoz C, Arevalo M, et al. Functional capacity of colostral leukocytes from women delivering prematurely. J Pediatr Gastroenterol Nutr 1989; 8(1):89–94.

43. Mehta R, Petrova A. Biologically active breast milk proteins in association with very preterm delivery and stage of lactation. J Perinatol 2011;31(1):58–62.

44. Garofalo R. Cytokines in human milk. J Pediatr 2010;156(Suppl 2):S36–40.
45. Saarinen UM, Kajosaari M. Breastfeeding as prophylaxis against atopic disease: prospective follow-up study until 17 years old. Lancet 1995;346(8982): 1065–9.
46. Koletzko S, Sherman P, Corey M, et al. Role of infant feeding practices in development of Crohn's disease in childhood. BMJ 1989;298(6688):1617–8.
47. Mayer EJ, Hamman RF, Gay EC, et al. Reduced risk of IDDM among breast-fed children. The Colorado IDDM Registry. Diabetes 1988;37(12):1625–32.
48. Walker A. Breast milk as the gold standard for protective nutrients. J Pediatr 2010;156(Suppl 2):S3–7.
49. McCracken VJ, Lorenz RG. The gastrointestinal ecosystem: a precarious alliance among epithelium, immunity and microbiota. Cell Microbiol 2001;3(1):1–11.
50. Walker WA. Initial intestinal colonization in the human infant and immune homeostasis. Ann Nutr Metab 2013;63(Suppl 2):8–15.
51. Collier-Hyams LS, Sloane V, Batten BC, et al. Cutting edge: bacterial modulation of epithelial signaling via changes in neddylation of cullin-1. J Immunol 2005; 175(7):4194–8.
52. Hooper LV, Wong MH, Thelin A, et al. Molecular analysis of commensal host-microbial relationships in the intestine. Science 2001;291(5505):881–4.
53. Kelly D, Campbell JI, King TP, et al. Commensal anaerobic gut bacteria attenuate inflammation by regulating nuclear-cytoplasmic shuttling of PPAR-gamma and RelA. Nat Immunol 2004;5(1):104–12.
54. Tao Y, Drabik KA, Waypa TS, et al. Soluble factors from *Lactobacillus* GG activate MAPKs and induce cytoprotective heat shock proteins in intestinal epithelial cells. Am J Physiol Cell Physiol 2006;290(4):C1018–30.
55. Yan F, Polk DB. Probiotic bacterium prevents cytokine-induced apoptosis in intestinal epithelial cells. J Biol Chem 2002;277(52):50959–65.
56. Mirpuri J, Brazil JC, Berardinelli AJ, et al. Commensal *Escherichia coli* reduces epithelial apoptosis through IFN-alphaA-mediated induction of guanylate binding protein-1 in human and murine models of developing intestine. J Immunol 2010;184(12):7186–95.
57. Rimoldi M, Chieppa M, Salucci V, et al. Intestinal immune homeostasis is regulated by the crosstalk between epithelial cells and dendritic cells. Nat Immunol 2005;6(5):507–14.
58. Yoshioka H, Iseki K, Fujita K. Development and differences of intestinal flora in the neonatal period in breast-fed and bottle-fed infants. Pediatrics 1983;72(3): 317–21.
59. Newburg DS. Neonatal protection by an innate immune system of human milk consisting of oligosaccharides and glycans. J Anim Sci 2009;87(Suppl 13): 26–34.
60. McVeagh P, Miller JB. Human milk oligosaccharides: only the breast. J Paediatr Child Health 1997;33(4):281–6.
61. Insoft RM, Sanderson IR, Walker WA. Development of immune function in the intestine and its role in neonatal diseases. Pediatr Clin North Am 1996;43(2): 551–71.
62. Newburg DS. Oligosaccharides and glycoconjugates in human milk: their role in host defense. J Mammary Gland Biol Neoplasia 1996;1(3):271–83.
63. Brandtzaeg P. The mucosal immune system and its integration with the mammary glands. J Pediatr 2010;156(Suppl 2):S8–15.
64. Xanthou M, Bines J, Walker WA. Human milk and intestinal host defense in newborns: an update. Adv Pediatr 1995;42:171–208.

65. Hanson LA. Comparative immunological studies of the immune globulins of human milk and of blood serum. Int Arch Allergy Appl Immunol 1961;18:241–67.
66. Newburg DS, Walker WA. Protection of the neonate by the innate immune system of developing gut and of human milk. Pediatr Res 2007;61(1):2–8.
67. Adamkin DH. Mother's milk, feeding strategies, and lactoferrin to prevent necrotizing enterocolitis. JPEN J Parenter Enteral Nutr 2012;36(Suppl 1):25S–9S.
68. Manzoni P, Rinaldi M, Cattani S, et al. Bovine lactoferrin supplementation for prevention of late-onset sepsis in very low-birth-weight neonates: a randomized trial. JAMA 2009;302(13):1421–8.
69. Manzoni P, Stolfi I, Messner H, et al. Bovine lactoferrin prevents invasive fungal infections in very low birth weight infants: a randomized controlled trial. Pediatrics 2012;129(1):116–23.
70. Valenti P, Antonini G. Lactoferrin: an important host defence against microbial and viral attack. Cell Mol Life Sci 2005;62(22):2576–87.
71. Kuwata H, Yip TT, Tomita M, et al. Direct evidence of the generation in human stomach of an antimicrobial peptide domain (lactoferricin) from ingested lactoferrin. Biochim Biophys Acta 1998;1429(1):129–41.
72. Ellison RT 3rd, Giehl TJ. Killing of gram-negative bacteria by lactoferrin and lysozyme. J Clin Invest 1991;88(4):1080–91.
73. Sherman MP. Lactoferrin and necrotizing enterocolitis. Clin Perinatol 2013;40(1): 79–91.
74. Mulligan P, White NR, Monteleone G, et al. Breast milk lactoferrin regulates gene expression by binding bacterial DNA CpG motifs but not genomic DNA promoters in model intestinal cells. Pediatr Res 2006;59(5):656–61.
75. Manzoni P, Mostert M, Stronati M. Lactoferrin for prevention of neonatal infections. Curr Opin Infect Dis 2011;24(3):177–82.
76. Buccigrossi V, de Marco G, Bruzzese E, et al. Lactoferrin induces concentration-dependent functional modulation of intestinal proliferation and differentiation. Pediatr Res 2007;61(4):410–4.
77. Haversen L, Ohlsson BG, Hahn-Zoric M, et al. Lactoferrin down-regulates the LPS-induced cytokine production in monocytic cells via NF-kappa B. Cell Immunol 2002;220(2):83–95.
78. Lonnerdal B. Bioactive proteins in breast milk. J Paediatr Child Health 2013; 49(Suppl 1):1–7.
79. Plaisancie P, Claustre J, Estienne M, et al. A novel bioactive peptide from yoghurts modulates expression of the gel-forming MUC2 mucin as well as population of goblet cells and Paneth cells along the small intestine. J Nutr Biochem 2013;24(1):213–21.
80. Lonnerdal B. Bioactive proteins in human milk: mechanisms of action. J Pediatr 2010;156(Suppl 2):S26–30.
81. Newburg DS. Do the binding properties of oligosaccharides in milk protect human infants from gastrointestinal bacteria? J Nutr 1997;127(Suppl 5): 980S–4S.
82. Stromqvist M, Falk P, Bergstrom S, et al. Human milk kappa-casein and inhibition of *Helicobacter pylori* adhesion to human gastric mucosa. J Pediatr Gastroenterol Nutr 1995;21(3):288–96.
83. Claud EC, Savidge T, Walker WA. Modulation of human intestinal epithelial cell IL-8 secretion by human milk factors. Pediatr Res 2003;53(3):419–25.
84. Neu J, Mihatsch WA, Zegarra J, et al. Intestinal mucosal defense system, Part 1. Consensus recommendations for immunonutrients. J Pediatr 2013;162(Suppl 3): S56–63.

85. Garofalo R, Chheda S, Mei F, et al. Interleukin-10 in human milk. Pediatr Res 1995;37(4 Pt 1):444–9.
86. Kuhn R, Lohler J, Rennick D, et al. Interleukin-10-deficient mice develop chronic enterocolitis. Cell 1993;75(2):263–74.
87. Glocker EO, Kotlarz D, Boztug K, et al. Inflammatory bowel disease and mutations affecting the interleukin-10 receptor. N Engl J Med 2009;361(21):2033–45.
88. Emami CN, Chokshi N, Wang J, et al. Role of interleukin-10 in the pathogenesis of necrotizing enterocolitis. Am J Surg 2012;203(4):428–35.
89. Dvorak B, Halpern MD, Holubec H, et al. Maternal milk reduces severity of necrotizing enterocolitis and increases intestinal IL-10 in a neonatal rat model. Pediatr Res 2003;53(3):426–33.
90. Penttila IA. Milk-derived transforming growth factor-beta and the infant immune response. J Pediatr 2010;156(Suppl 2):S21–5.
91. Chang M, Suen Y, Lee SM, et al. Transforming growth factor-beta 1, macrophage inflammatory protein-1 alpha, and interleukin-8 gene expression is lower in stimulated human neonatal compared with adult mononuclear cells. Blood 1994;84(1):118–24.
92. Hawkes JS, Bryan DL, James MJ, et al. Cytokines (IL-1beta, IL-6, TNF-alpha, TGF-beta1, and TGF-beta2) and prostaglandin E2 in human milk during the first three months postpartum. Pediatr Res 1999;46(2):194–9.
93. Kalliomaki M, Ouwehand A, Arvilommi H, et al. Transforming growth factor-beta in breast milk: a potential regulator of atopic disease at an early age. J Allergy Clin Immunol 1999;104(6):1251–7.
94. Oddy WH, Halonen M, Martinez FD, et al. TGF-beta in human milk is associated with wheeze in infancy. J Allergy Clin Immunol 2003;112(4):723–8.
95. Ogawa J, Sasahara A, Yoshida T, et al. Role of transforming growth factor-beta in breast milk for initiation of IgA production in newborn infants. Early Hum Dev 2004;77(1–2):67–75.
96. Dvorak B. Milk epidermal growth factor and gut protection. J Pediatr 2010; 156(Suppl 2):S31–5.
97. Dvorak B, Fituch CC, Williams CS, et al. Increased epidermal growth factor levels in human milk of mothers with extremely premature infants. Pediatr Res 2003;54(1):15–9.
98. Coursodon CF, Dvorak B. Epidermal growth factor and necrotizing enterocolitis. Curr Opin Pediatr 2012;24(2):160–4.
99. Dvorak B, Halpern MD, Holubec H, et al. Epidermal growth factor reduces the development of necrotizing enterocolitis in a neonatal rat model. Am J Physiol Gastrointest Liver Physiol 2002;282(1):G156–64.
100. Clark JA, Doelle SM, Halpern MD, et al. Intestinal barrier failure during experimental necrotizing enterocolitis: protective effect of EGF treatment. Am J Physiol Gastrointest Liver Physiol 2006;291(5):G938–49.
101. Ichikawa M, Sugita M, Takahashi M, et al. Breast milk macrophages spontaneously produce granulocyte-macrophage colony-stimulating factor and differentiate into dendritic cells in the presence of exogenous interleukin-4 alone. Immunology 2003;108(2):189–95.
102. Thormar H, Isaacs CE, Brown HR, et al. Inactivation of enveloped viruses and killing of cells by fatty acids and monoglycerides. Antimicrob Agents Chemother 1987;31(1):27–31.

Donor Human Milk for Preterm Infants

What It Is, What It Can Do, and What Still Needs to Be Learned

Tarah T. Colaizy, MD, MPH

KEYWORDS

- Donor human milk • VLBW infant • Necrotizing enterocolitis
- Neurodevelopmental outcomes

KEY POINTS

- Donor human milk is different from maternal milk, and although similar or equivalent benefits might be postulated, high-quality evidence for benefits of donor milk use in very low birth weight (VLBW) infants in the era of routine human milk fortification is sparse.
- There is a significant body of evidence that maternal human milk use results in superior outcomes in multiple domains (infection, neurodevelopment) compared with formula diets in VLBW infants.
- Donor milk is an appropriate choice for VLBW infants whose maternal milk is either insufficient in quantity or unavailable.

INTRODUCTION

Donor human milk is not a new idea, with wet-nursing being a common practice for all of recorded history. The Code of Hammurabi, written in 1770 BC, outlines punishment for wet-nurses whose charges die,[1] and Soranus laid out ideal attributes for wet nurses in first century AD Rome.[2] Milk banking began in France in the 1800s, with the first human milk bank formed in the United States in Boston, Massachusetts, in 1912. In 1934, the Dionne quintuplets were fed an estimated 237 L (8000 oz) of milk donated by women from Toronto, which was shipped to their rural Ontario home by train.[3]

As evidence of differences in outcomes of very low birth weight (VLBW) infants fed maternal human milk compared with those fed infant formula has mounted, donor human milk has become an increasingly used intervention when maternal milk is unavailable. Use of maternal milk during the birth hospitalization in VLBW infants has been

Carver College of Medicine, Department of Pediatrics, University of Iowa, 200 Hawkins Drive, 8809 JPP, Iowa City, IA 52242, USA
E-mail address: tarah-colaizy@uiowa.edu

Clin Perinatol 41 (2014) 437–450
http://dx.doi.org/10.1016/j.clp.2014.02.003
0095-5108/14/$ – see front matter © 2014 Elsevier Inc. All rights reserved.
perinatology.theclinics.com

associated with lessened in-hospital morbidity including lower rates of necrotizing enterocolitis (NEC),[4–8] late-onset sepsis,[4,5] bronchopulmonary dysplasia,[4,9] the composite outcome of NEC or death,[10] and severe retinopathy of prematurity.[7] Maternal milk diets have also been associated with shorter hospital stays[4] and lower incidence of rehospitalization[9] than preterm formula diets. Most important for lifelong benefit, maternal milk intake in preterm infants has also been associated with superior neurodevelopmental outcomes compared with formula diets, measured at 18 to 22 months,[9] 30 months,[11] and 7 to 8 years,[12] with demonstration of a significant dose-response relationship.[9,12]

Donor human milk, dispensed as a pooled, pasteurized product from accredited milk banks, is used as a replacement for infant formula when maternal milk is insufficient or unavailable to the VLBW infant. Most donor human milk dispensed in the United States and Canada to preterm infants comes from the member banks of the Human Milk Banking Association of North America (HMBANA). Growth in milk banking in North America has been brisk over the past decade, with 6 banks dispensing in 2003 and 16 in 2013, with 3 more in the development phase. In 2011, the member banks of the HMBANA dispensed more than 64,470 L (2.18 million ounces) of donor milk, up from 32,530 L (1.1 million ounces) dispensed in 2007.[13] Donor milk is also available commercially, from Prolacta Bioscience (Monrovia, CA).

Donor human milk is different from maternal milk, and although similar or equivalent benefits might be postulated, high-quality evidence for benefits of donor milk use in VLBW infants in the era of routine human milk fortification is sparse.

This article introduces donor human milk and describes the known biological differences between maternal milk and donor milk. Evidence for benefits of donor human milk for VLBW infants compared with term or preterm infant formula is explored.

DONOR MILK: AN INTRODUCTION

Donor human milk dispensed by milk banks is obtained in North America from volunteer donors, most of whom have given birth to healthy term infants. Donors may donate existing frozen stored milk, may express milk in an ongoing manner specifically for donation to the bank, or may use a combination of these donation strategies. Milk donors undergo a thorough screening process to assess for behavioral risk factors for blood-borne infection, and undergo serologic screening for all strains of human immunodeficiency virus (HIV), HTLV I and II (Human T-Lymphocytic Virus), hepatitis B and C, and syphilis. They may not be users of nicotine products or use alcohol daily in excess of 2 drinks. Few chronic medications are compatible with milk donation, with only low-dose oral contraceptives, insulin, thyroid hormone replacement, and selected selective serotonin reuptake inhibitors allowed. Medications taken for temporary periods require abstaining from milk donation for 5 times the half-life of the medication,[14] and donors are instructed to refrain from expressing milk for donation within 12 hours following alcohol consumption.[14]

Donor Milk Processing

Donors express milk at home, using personally owned equipment. They are given instruction on clean technique for milk expression, including cleaning of pump parts, hand washing, appropriate storage containers, and handling of milk. Milk is stored frozen before delivery to the milk bank. At the bank, frozen milk from several donors is thawed gradually in refrigerators. It is pooled to equilibrate the nutritional content of the milk. Donor milk in North America is then pasteurized by one of 2 methods: Holder pasteurization or high-temperature short-time (HTST) pasteurization. Member banks of HMBANA use the Holder method, in which sealed bottles of pooled milk are heated in a water bath to 62°C and maintained at that temperature for 30 minutes. The HTST procedure used by Prolacta Bioscience uses a temperature of 72°C for 16 seconds.[15] Milk is then quickly chilled in an ice bath and frozen at −20°C until dispensed. A bottle from each batch is sent for bacteriologic testing and must contain less than 1 cfu/mL of bacteria to qualify for dispensing.[14]

Pasteurization and Effects on Human Milk

The good: prevention of bacterial and viral disease transmission
In North America, donor milk is pasteurized to reduce or eliminate the risk of transmission of bacterial and viral disease to recipients. Bacterial colonization of milk donated to milk banks is common. All raw milk donated to the Mother's Milk Bank of Texas in 2003 was subjected to bacterial culture, both as individual donor samples and as pool samples. Milk from 78% of mothers grew at least one organism, and most pooled samples grew at least 2 organisms. Eighty-seven percent of pooled samples grew coagulase-negative *Staphylococcus*, and 61% grew at least one gram-negative organism.[16] Holder pasteurization eradicated most bacteria, because 93% of pooled samples were sterile on postpasteurization culture.[16] The HTST pasteurization procedure has also been shown to eradicate colonization of donor milk contaminated by *Escherichia coli*, *Staphylococcus aureus*, and *Staphylococcus agalactiae* under experimental conditions.[15] In a more recent study comparing bacterial profiles of Internet-sourced informally shared milk and donor bank samples, 20 donor samples from the Ohio Mother's Milk Bank had a 35% colonization rate with gram-negative organisms, 25% coliform organisms, 25% *Staphylococcus* spp, and 20% *Streptococcus* spp; 25% had no bacterial colonization.[17] Viral colonization of donor milk also occurs. A study of Norwegian milk donors reported that 62% of donors were cytomegalovirus (CMV) immunoglobulin (Ig) G positive,[18] although milk was not tested for the presence of CMV. In the previously discussed study of informally shared versus donor-banked milk, 5% of milk bank samples similarly tested positive for CMV, and none positive for HIV.[17] Both Holder and HTST procedures have been shown to eradicate CMV infectivity in vitro.[19]

The bad: impact on anti-infectious properties of donor human milk
Although pasteurization protects donor milk recipients, it also negatively affects some of the unique anti-infectious properties of human milk. Human milk contains active maternal T cells,[20] B cells, macrophages, and neutrophils,[21] all of which are inactivated by pasteurization.[22] In addition, secretory IgA levels are reduced by 28% to 60% with Holder pasteurization,[23–25] and lactoferrin and lysozyme activity are reduced up to 80% and 60%, respectively.[25] Pasteurization does not affect the levels of human milk oligosaccharides,[26] and although patterns and levels of these compounds may differ between donor and maternal milk fed to VLBW infants in neonatal intensive care units (NICUs),[27] the significance of this is unclear.

Nutritional Properties of Donor Human Milk Versus Maternal Milk

Donor milk differs nutritionally from maternal milk to some degree when fed to VLBW infants, and neonatologists should be aware of these differences because they may affect the need for nutrient fortification when donor milk is used. Some of these differences are consequences of pasteurization, but others are simply a result of handling of donor milk and stage of lactation of donors compared with mothers of newborn VLBW infants. Most studies report that pasteurization does not affect protein, fat, and carbohydrate levels of human milk[23,28] but a recent study of Brazilian banked milk refuted this, showing modest decreases in protein (6%) and fat (8%) when milk was pasteurized, frozen, and thawed.[29] Levels of most vitamins and minerals are not affected by pasteurization,[30,31] although milk antioxidant capacity is significantly reduced, more so with Holder compared with HTST methods,[32] which could be hypothesized to affect infection preventative actions of human milk.

Protein content of donor human milk approaches the generally accepted standard estimate of 1 g/dL for term human milk,[33] but typically does not reach the levels of 1.2 to 1.5 g/dL reported for milk expressed by mothers delivering preterm in the first 4 to 6 weeks after delivery.[34] This is a consequence not of pasteurization but of donors donating later in lactation after having delivered term infants. In a study of a US nationwide sample of donor milk, mean protein content was 1.16 g/dL, but 30% of the 415 samples tested contained less than 1 g/dL,[33] and a study of 1 year of milk donations to the Mother's Milk Bank of Iowa reported mean protein content of donated milk to be 0.85 g/dL.[35] A study of samples from the Mother's Milk Bank of Ohio similarly reported a mean protein content of 0.9 g/dl[28] with only minor before-and-after pasteurization differences in free amino acid concentrations. Fat content of donor milk is reported to be 3.22 to 3.9 g/dL for pooled samples, similar to that for preterm maternal milk, with similar wide variability,[33–35] although there is a higher concentration of free fatty acids in pasteurized milk than in fresh milk.[36]

Long-chain Polyunsaturated Fatty Acid Levels in Donor Human Milk

Levels of the long-chain polyunsaturated fatty acids (LC-PUFAs) docosahexaenoic acid (DHA) and arachidonic acid (ARA) vary among milk samples from different milk banks, and are often less than the reported US mean DHA concentration of 0.14%.[37,38] Holder pasteurization did not significantly change the concentration of these molecules in human milk samples, but samples obtained from the Mother's Milk Bank of Iowa contained a mean concentration of DHA of only 0.07%, much lower than reported nationwide levels. Milk from several other geographically diverse HMBANA banks contained levels similar to reported US means, including Texas, North Carolina, and California.[37] The investigators hypothesized that donors in the Midwest are less likely to consume dietary LC-PUFAs in the form of fatty fish than are donors nearer coastal areas. This difference may need to be considered when using donor human milk, particularly when DHA content is compared with the levels with which infant formula is supplemented, which are higher (0.14%–0.32%, depending on product).

Current State of the Evidence: Differences Between Maternal and Donor Milk

- Pasteurization results in inactivation of white blood cells, bacteria, and viruses in human milk.
- Pasteurization also results in loss of some protective compounds present in milk, whereas others are not affected.
- Donor milk obtained from term donors contains less fat and protein than typical preterm maternal milk, and may not contain adequate DHA and ARA.
- Differences between maternal and donor milk should be recognized and addressed when donor milk is fed to VLBW infants.

OUTCOMES OF VLBW INFANTS FED DONOR HUMAN MILK COMPARED WITH OTHER DIETS
NEC

Maternal human milk compared with formula diets has been shown to be consistently protective against NEC in VLBW infants in multiple studies conducted over the past

30 years,[4–7,10] when fed with or without multicomponent fortifiers.[4–8,10] It is reasonable to think that donor human milk would perform similarly, and limited evidence suggests that this is the case. Several trials of unfortified donor human milk compared with formula diets were performed in the 1980s, and 2 high-quality meta-analyses including these trials have been published.[39,40] Boyd and colleagues[39] conducted a meta-analysis of 3 trials of preterm infants born in the 1970s and 1980s[41,42] that were designed to compare growth between infants fed diets of contemporary preterm formulas and infants fed unfortified donor human milk. Two of the studies were randomized,[6,42] and 1 was observational.[41] NEC was reported as a secondary outcome in all studies, and was not statistically significantly associated with either diet in any of the trials. When meta-analysis was performed, the donor human milk diet was associated with significantly lower risk of NEC (combined relative risk [RR], 0.21; 95% confidence interval [CI], 0.06–0.76; $P = .017$). Stated another way, an unfortified donor human milk diet reduced the risk of NEC by 79% (95% CI, 24%, 94%). The investigators calculated that, in populations in which the risk of NEC in formula-fed infants is 5% to 20%, 18.5 (95% CI, 9.7–200) preterm infants would have to be fed donor milk to prevent 1 case of NEC.[39] Quigley and colleagues[40] performed another high-quality meta-analysis of trials comparing a variety of donor milk diets with preterm formula diets. Two trials selected for the Boyd and colleagues[6] meta-analysis described earlier were also included in the analysis of formula (all types) compared with unfortified donor human milk as the sole diet,[6,42] as well as an additional small randomized trial from the same time period.[43] Analysis of these 3 trials yielded an RR of 0.25 (95% CI, 0.06, 0.98; $P = .047$) for development of NEC with donor milk diets, which is a similar effect size to that noted earlier.[40]

Although these data are intriguing, they are difficult to interpret when choosing a diet for contemporary VLBW infants whose mothers' milk is not available or is available in insufficient quantity. Rates of breastfeeding initiation have recently been high in mothers of VLBW infants,[44] but mother's milk alone is often insufficient,[45] so a more typical diet consists of partial maternal milk and partial formula or donor human milk. In addition, all types of human milk fed to VLBW infants are routinely fortified with multicomponent human milk fortifiers (HMFs), rather than being unmodified as in the trials that comprise the meta-analyses described earlier. There is limited additional evidence regarding fortified donor human milk use in practice. Schanler and colleagues[5] published the first randomized trial of fortified donor human milk compared with preterm formula as a supplement to maternal milk in 2005, in which NEC was reported as a primary outcome. Bovine milk–derived fortifier was used in this trial. VLBW infants whose mothers intended to provide maternal milk were randomized to receive donor human milk or preterm formula if maternal milk supply was insufficient. Infants receiving only a fortified maternal milk diet and those receiving donor milk supplements experienced the lowest incidence of NEC (6% in both groups), with a higher incidence in the group supplemented with preterm formula (11%), although these differences were not statistically significant ($P = .27$, donor milk vs formula; $P = .39$, maternal milk vs both supplement groups combined).

Recent evidence suggests that combined use of both donor human milk and human milk–derived HMF (HHMF), both as supplements to maternal milk when insufficient,[46] and as a sole diet when mothers decline to initiate breastfeeding[47] results in lower NEC incidence than using preterm formula in these circumstances. This dietary approach, referred to as the exclusive human milk diet (EHM), is now possible because of commercial availability of HHMF. Sullivan and colleagues[46] randomized VLBW infants whose mothers were providing milk to receive either the EHM diet (donor milk as a supplement if maternal milk insufficient plus HHMF for all human milk), or a diet containing all available maternal milk, fortified with bovine milk–derived HMF (BHMF), and supplemented with preterm infant formula if maternal milk insufficient. Infants in EHM group experienced a lower rate of NEC, both medical and surgical. The odds ratio for NEC with the EHM diet was estimated as 0.23 (95% CI, 0.08, 0.66; P = .007) relative to the diet containing BHMF and/or preterm formula. All infants in this trial who developed surgical NEC received BHMF or formula, either by trial design or by protocol violation. Cristofalo and colleagues[47] studied the EHM diet in the setting of mothers who never provide milk to their infants, randomizing 53 VLBW infants to a sole EHM diet or a sole diet of preterm formula for the duration of hospitalization. NEC occurred in only 1 infant in the EHM group (3%), but in 5 infants in the formula group (21%; P = .08).

Current State of the Evidence: NEC and Donor Milk

- The most common mode of donor milk use (ie, as a supplement to maternal milk with BHMF) is poorly studied with regard to risk of NEC compared with formula supplementation, but such use may be protective.
- NEC risk of donor milk plus BHMF as a sole diet has not been compared with the risk with preterm formula.
- The EHM diet shows promise as an intervention that may be superior to formula use; both sole formula diets and maternal milk diets supplemented with formula.

Growth in VLBW Infants Fed Donor Human Milk

VLBW infants fed unfortified[48] and fortified[4,49] maternal milk have been consistently reported to grow more slowly in early life than those fed preterm or term formula, which is concerning because poor growth in this period has been associated with potentially lifelong neurodevelopmental impairment.[50] Several investigations of growth in preterm infants fed donor human milk have been undertaken, both with unfortified and fortified donor human milk. Multiple trials of in-hospital growth of infants fed unfortified donor milk and the only trial of fortified donor milk[5] compared with term or preterm formulas were reviewed for the Cochrane Report in 2007, with growth outcomes analyzed for studies of donor milk as both a sole diet and a supplement to maternal milk.[40] In the sole diet category, only studies of unfortified donor milk were available, and infants fed donor milk grew 2.7 g/kg/d (95% CI, 2.0, 3.4) slower than those fed formula. Two studies of donor milk supplementation to maternal milk, 1 unfortified,[48] and 1 fortified,[5] were combined for analysis, and a similar growth deficit was noted: infants fed donor milk grew 2.4 g/kg/d (95% CI, 1.3, 3.5) more slowly. When all trials, sole diet and supplemental, were combined for analysis, the growth deficit was similar (2.59 g/kg/d; 95% CI, 1.99, 3.2).[40] Again, most of the trials included in these meta-analyses used unfortified donor milk, which is not a currently used diet in VLBW infants. Therefore, the ability to generalize these results to current clinical practice is limited.

Two trials have reported in-hospital growth in infants fed bovine-fortified donor human milk both as a supplement to maternal milk and as a sole diet. One reported growth as a secondary outcome.[5] Infants fed donor milk supplement gained weight more slowly than those fed formula supplements, with a deficit of 3 g/kg/d (P = .001), but length and head circumference growth was similar between groups. Infants fed donor milk grew similarly to those fed solely maternal milk in this trial (difference, 1.7 g/kg/d in favor of maternal milk; P = .08).[5] Colaizy and colleagues[51] studied growth by amount and type of bovine-fortified human milk received by a cohort of VLBW infants born between 2003 and 2005. Most of the infants received more than 75% human milk throughout hospitalization, with varying proportions of donor and maternal milk.

Although diets with more than 75% human milk compared with diets containing less human milk were associated with a larger negative change in weight z score from birth to discharge (-0.6 vs -0.3; $P = .03$), type of human milk was not significantly associated with z-score change. Infants receiving more than 75% of the in-hospital diet as donor milk experienced a weight z-score change of -0.84 versus -0.56 for infants receiving more than 75% maternal milk ($P = .28$). Infants in this trial also received levels of protein fortification in excess of those produced with manufacturer-directed BHMF use, through additional BHMF use or as single-component protein powders.[51]

Three trials have reported growth outcomes for infants fed the EHM diet: the 2 multicenter interventional trials discussed earlier regarding NEC,[46,47] and an additional single-center observational trial.[52] In the trial comparing a diet of maternal milk fortified with BHMF and supplemented with formula versus a diet of maternal milk fortified with HHMF and supplemented with donor milk, infants gained weight similarly in both groups (14.2 g/kg/d human group vs 15.1 g/kg/d bovine group; $P = .13$).[46] Length and head circumference gain were also similar between diet groups in this study. In the subsequent study comparing the EHM diet with a diet of preterm formula in infants whose mothers did not provide milk, rate of weight gain was similar between groups (17 g/kg/d for bovine group vs 15 g/kg/d for human milk group; $P>.05$), but infants in the bovine group experienced faster length gain (1.12 cm/wk vs 0.84 cm/wk in the human group; $P = .006$). Head circumference gain was similar between groups (0.88 cm/wk in the bovine group vs 0.78 cm/wk in the human group).[47] A single-center observational trial was conducted after institution of EHM for infants less than 1250 g at birth, fed EHM through 34 weeks postmenstrual age (PMA).[52] The investigators used an aggressive early fortification scheme, with all infants receiving HHMF to fortify their maternal or donor milk to 36.4 KJ/dL (26 kcal/oz), similar to the bovine-based strategy reported by Colaizy and colleagues.[51] With this feeding regimen, rates of growth were better than typically reported for infants fed human milk, regardless of fortifier type. Weight gain was 24.8 g/kg/d from birth to 34 weeks PMA, length gain was 0.99 cm/wk, and head circumference growth was 0.72 cm/wk. The investigators compared these values with those reported for the first trial of the EHM diet[46] and noted better weight gain ($P<.0001$), better length gain ($P = .008$), and similar head circumference gain ($P = .84$).

Current State of the Evidence: Growth in VLBW Infants Fed Donor Human Milk

- VLBW infants fed human milk are typically reported to grow more slowly during birth hospitalization than those fed formula, when both maternal and donor milk are studied.
- Recent studies report improved rates of growth with dietary strategies that focus on protein supplementation beyond standard fortifier use according to manufacturer recommendations.
- These strategies should be used, or neonatologists should at least be aware that additional protein supplementation may be needed in VBLW infants fed donor human milk.

Length of Hospital Stay, Length of Parenteral Nutrition

Maternal human milk feeding in VLBW infants has been shown to decrease length of initial hospital stay, as well as length of parenteral nutrition use. Schanler and colleagues[4] reported that hospital stay was shortened by 15 days, and total parenteral nutrition (TPN) use decreased by 10 days when fortified maternal milk was fed compared with preterm formula. Both of these outcomes result in substantial cost savings to the medical system, and in 2001 Wight[53] estimated the cost savings of using donor human milk using the effect size estimates from these data. She calculated that $10,600 2001 dollars could be saved per infant in hospital daily charges and TPN cost by using donor milk. However, this figure assumes that use of donor human milk in lieu of formula results in the same outcomes as maternal milk use, which has not been thoroughly investigated.

Hospital length of stay and TPN use length have been studied for donor milk used as a supplement to maternal milk, and in both studies of the EHM diet. Schanler and colleagues'[5] study of donor milk as a supplement to maternal milk compared length of stay in donor milk supplemented infants with those supplemented with preterm formula and found no difference (87 days for donor milk vs 90 days for preterm formula; $P = .66$). However, the control infants fed entirely with maternal milk experienced shorter stays (75 days; $P = .04$ vs both supplements), suggesting that donor milk may not be as effective as maternal milk in reducing length of stay. Although the investigators did not study length of TPN use specifically, they reported length of central venous catheter use, which can be used as a surrogate for TPN use. Infants in all three groups had similar length of central catheter use.

When the EHM diet was studied in VLBW infants receiving maternal milk, infants who received formula supplements and bovine fortifier experienced similar length of stay to those receiving the EHM diet ($P = .9$), and length of TPN use also did not vary by type of supplement and fortifier ($P = .71$).[46] However, when the EHM diet was studied as an alternative to formula for VLBW infants whose mothers never provided milk, infants receiving human milk received fewer days of TPN (28 days EHM vs 36 days formula; $P = .04$), and were hospitalized for 10 fewer days than those fed formula, although the difference in length of stay was not significant.[47]

Current State of the Evidence: Donor Human Milk and Hospital Stay, TPN Use

- Donor human milk, fortified with bovine fortifier and used as a supplement to maternal milk, has not been shown to affect TPN usage or length of hospital stay
- Donor human milk, fortified with human HMF and used as a supplement to maternal milk, has not been shown to affect length of stay or TPN use compared with the use of bovine fortifier and formula supplements to maternal milk
- An EHM diet is associated with shorter length of TPN use compared with preterm formula in infants receiving no maternal milk

Neurodevelopmental Outcomes

The most significant benefits of maternal human milk feeding in VLBW infants arguably are neurodevelopmental advantages. Similar to evidence in term infants,[54] several investigators have reported that VLBW infants fed maternal milk during the birth hospitalization have higher neurodevelopmental testing scores at age 18 to 22 months,[9] 30 months,[11] and 7 to 8 years.[12] In the cohort studied by Vohr and colleagues,[11] in which neurodevelopmental benefits persisted to 30 months in extremely low birth weight (ELBW) infants fed human milk, and in which a dose-response relationship was identified between volume of milk fed and Bayley Scales of Infant Development II scores, these benefits were similar for infants fed maternal milk only during hospitalization as well as in those who were subsequently breastfed at home. This finding is compelling, because it suggests that a dietary intervention given for a few months in infancy can result in lifelong functional benefit. However, it is not known whether donor human milk results in similar developmental advantages.

Women who breastfeed in the United States tend to be older, better educated, and have higher incomes than those who do not,[44] and these characteristics are also associated with better neurodevelopmental outcomes for preterm infants. In a study undertaken in the Netherlands of former VLBW infants, intelligence quotient (IQ) at age 19 years was most strongly associated with parental education, with children of highly educated parents scoring 14.2 points higher in IQ than children of parents with low educational achievement. This difference in IQ by parental education was more pronounced than the effect of any other variable studied, including gestational age and in utero growth retardation status.[55] Thus, maternal breastfeeding may be a surrogate measure for an enriched environment, and some of the effect seen with improved neurodevelopmental outcomes with maternal milk feeding of ELBWs may not be caused by the human milk, but rather by the mother. Donor human milk isolates the effect of the milk from the effects of social factors associated with breastfeeding.

There have been 2 studies of neurodevelopmental outcomes in preterm infants fed donor human milk, both of which were performed with unfortified donor human milk. Lucas and colleagues[56] published a randomized controlled trial of donor milk and neurodevelopmental outcomes in preterm infants, undertaken in the United Kingdom in the 1980s. Infants less than 1850 g at birth whose mothers did not provide milk were randomized to unfortified donor milk or preterm formula diets during hospitalization, and their neurodevelopmental outcomes were assessed using the Bayley Scales of Infant Development II at 18 to 22 months of age. Developmental outcomes in the two groups were similar but, when the outcomes in infants fed donor milk were compared with outcomes in another cohort, studied by the same investigators, who were fed term formula, donor milk was associated with neurodevelopmental advantage. Infants fed donor milk scored 8.8 points higher on the Bayley Mental Development Index, and 2.1 points higher on the Bayley Psychomotor Development Index than did those fed term formula. A similar study was performed in the United States.[43] VLBW infants were randomized at 10 days of age to unfortified donor milk or term formula, and neurodevelopmental outcomes were assessed at 37 weeks PMA using the Brazelton Neonatal Behavioral Assessment Scale. Infants fed donor milk experienced significant growth failure compared with those fed formula, and performed more poorly on a task that tested orientation to inanimate stimuli ($P<.02$).[43] However, neither of these studies informs current practice well because unfortified milk is not routinely fed to VLBW infants. The infants who were fed unfortified donor milk in the large randomized trial by Lucas and colleagues[56] performed similarly to those fed preterm formula, despite experiencing higher rates of growth failure, suggesting that there are positive neurodevelopmental effects of human milk that are separate from maternal factors that can overcome the detrimental effects of poor growth.

At the time of this publication, there are 3 randomized trials of fortified donor human milk underway in VLBW infants, all of which were designed with neurodevelopmental outcome as the primary outcome. Two single-center trials, one in Canada (the Donor Milk for Improved Neurodevelopmental Outcomes [DoMINO] Trial, ISRCTN3531714) and one in the United States (Donor Human Milk and Neurodevelopmental Outcomes in VLBW Infants, clinicaltrials.gov NCT01232725), have randomized infants to receive fortified donor milk or preterm formula as a supplement to maternal milk, and are assessing outcomes at 18 to 22 months. A third trial, underway at the centers of the National Institute of Child Health and Human Development Neonatal Research Network (The MILK trial, NCT01534481), will randomize 670 infants whose mothers provide no or minimal milk to fortified donor breast milk or preterm formula, and will assess outcomes at 22 to 26 months. The results of these trials, which collectively will test this intervention in 1000 ELBW infants, should be instrumental in determining the developmental effects of donor milk.

Current State of the Evidence: Donor Human Milk and Neurodevelopmental Outcomes

- Neurodevelopmental effects of fortified donor human milk have not been studied, but 3 studies are underway.
- Unfortified donor milk has been shown to result in BSID II scores at 18 to 22 months that are superior to those of term formula in preterm infants.

PROFESSIONAL SOCIETY RECOMMENDATIONS

Two prominent professional bodies have recently published recommendations for the use of donor human milk in preterm infants. The American Academy of Pediatrics, Section on Breastfeeding, published an updated policy statement, *Breastfeeding and the Use of Human Milk*, in 2012. The statement recommends that all preterm infants receive maternal milk, or, if not available, that pasteurized donor milk should be used.[57] This statement cites the Cochrane Review[40] and the study of the EHM diet as a supplement to maternal milk,[46] both of which are extensively discussed earlier as evidence for this recommendation. The European Society for Pediatric Gastroenterology, Hepatology, and Nutrition Committee on Nutrition published a more extensive review of the use of donor human milk in preterm infants, and also recommends universal maternal milk feeding, with donor human milk as the preferred second-line diet.[58]

SUMMARY: SHOULD ALL VLBW INFANTS RECEIVE DONOR MILK IF MATERNAL MILK IS NOT AVAILABLE?

Donor human milk represents an intriguing option for the feeding of VLBW infants. There is a significant body of evidence that maternal human milk use results in superior outcomes in multiple domains (infection, neurodevelopment) compared with formula diets in VLBW infants. Clinicians should make extensive efforts to promote maternal provision of breast milk in NICUs, using lactation support, peer support, and environmental support (private room NICUs, provision of breast pumps, and so forth), all of which have been shown to improve the ability of mothers of VLBW infants to provide milk.

However, the optimal non–maternal-milk diet is yet to be determined. This article describes studies conducted during 2 eras of neonatal nutrition: before and after routine fortification of human milk in the VLBW population. In the unfortified era compared with various formula diets, donor milk has been associated with decreased risk of infectious complications of prematurity, poorer growth outcomes, and equivalent or improved neurodevelopmental outcomes. In the fortification era, bovine-fortified donor milk as a supplement to maternal milk has been associated with similar infectious complications and poorer growth outcomes to preterm formula. Human-fortified donor milk as a supplement to maternal milk, the EHM diet, has been associated with improved rates of NEC and poorer growth outcomes compared with bovine-fortified maternal milk supplemented with formula. In addition, human-fortified donor milk has been associated with lower rates of NEC and lower TPN usage compared with preterm formula in infants receiving no maternal milk. There are no published data regarding neurodevelopmental outcomes of infants receiving the EHM diet compared with a diet containing bovine fortifier and/or formula.

Where does this leave clinicians? In the limited studies available in the fortification era, donor milk has not been associated with adverse outcomes and there are hints of benefit, and the evidence from the unfortified era is more convincing as to benefit.

Therefore, donor milk is an appropriate choice for the VLBW infant whose maternal milk is either insufficient in quantity or unavailable. However, further research should be undertaken for this intervention, particularly in the areas of:

1. Neurodevelopmental outcomes of infants fed fortified donor milk compared with those fed formula
2. The impact of fortifier choice (bovine vs human) on growth, infectious outcomes, and neurodevelopmental outcomes

REFERENCES

1. The code of Hammurabi. Available at: http://avalon.law.yale.edu/subject_menus/hammenu.asp. Accessed December 2, 2013.
2. Advice on hiring a wet-nurse. In: Lefkowitz MR, Fant MB, editors. Women's life in Greece and Rome: a source book in translation. 1st edition. Baltimore (MD): The Johns Hopkins University Press; 2005. p. 268.
3. Arnold LD. Donor human milk for premature infants: the famous case of the Dionne quintuplets. J Hum Lact 1994;10(4):271–2.
4. Schanler RJ, Shulman RJ, Lau C. Feeding strategies for premature infants: beneficial outcomes of feeding fortified human milk versus preterm formula. Pediatrics 1999;103(6 Pt 1):1150–7.
5. Schanler RJ, Lau C, Hurst NM, et al. Randomized trial of donor human milk versus preterm formula as substitutes for mothers' own milk in the feeding of extremely premature infants. Pediatrics 2005;116(2):400–6.
6. Lucas A, Cole TJ. Breast milk and neonatal necrotising enterocolitis [see comment]. Lancet 1990;336(8730):1519–23.
7. Maayan-Metzger A, Avivi S, Schushan-Eisen I, et al. Human milk versus formula feeding among preterm infants: short-term outcomes. Am J Perinatol 2011;29:121–6.
8. Sisk PM, Lovelady CA, Dillard RG, et al. Early human milk feeding is associated with a lower risk of necrotizing enterocolitis in very low birth weight infants. J Perinatol 2007;27(7):428–33.
9. Vohr BR, Poindexter BB, Dusick AM, et al, for the NNRN. Beneficial effects of breast milk in the neonatal intensive care unit on the developmental outcome of extremely low birth weight infants at 18 months of age. Pediatrics 2006;118(1):e115–23.
10. Meinzen-Derr J, Poindexter B, Wrage L, et al. Role of human milk in extremely low birth weight infants' risk of necrotizing enterocolitis or death. J Perinatol 2009;29(1):57–62.
11. Vohr BR, Poindexter BB, Dusick AM, et al. Persistent beneficial effects of breast milk ingested in the neonatal intensive care unit on outcomes of extremely low birth weight infants at 30 months of age. Pediatrics 2007;120(4):e953–9.
12. Lucas A, Morley R, Cole TJ, et al. Breast milk and subsequent intelligence quotient in children born preterm [see comment]. Lancet 1992;339(8788):261–4.
13. HMBANA - who do we serve? Available at: http://www.hmbana.org/who-do-we-serve.
14. Human Milk Banking Association of North America. Guidelines for the establishment and operation of a donor human milk bank. Forth Worth, TX: Human Milk Banking Association of North America; 2011.
15. Terpstra FG, Rechtman DJ, Lee ML, et al. Antimicrobial and antiviral effect of high-temperature short-time (HTST) pasteurization applied to human milk. Breastfeed Med 2007;2(1):27–33.

16. Landers S, Updegrove K. Bacteriological screening of donor human milk before and after Holder pasteurization. Breastfeed Med 2010;5(3):117–21.

17. Keim SA, Hogan JS, McNamara KA, et al. Microbial contamination of human milk purchased via the internet. Pediatrics 2013;132(5):e1227–35.

18. Lindemann PC, Foshaugen I, Lindemann R. Characteristics of breast milk and serology of women donating breast milk to a milk bank. Arch Dis Child Fetal Neonatal Ed 2004;89(5):F440–1.

19. Hamprecht K, Maschmann J, Muller D, et al. Cytomegalovirus (CMV) inactivation in breast milk: reassessment of pasteurization and freeze-thawing. Pediatr Res 2004;56(4):529–35.

20. Wirt DP, Adkins LT, Palkowetz KH, et al. Activated and memory T lymphocytes in human milk. Cytometry 1992;13(3):282–90.

21. Field CJ. The immunological components of human milk and their effect on immune development in infants. J Nutr 2005;135(1):1–4.

22. Lawrence RA. Storage of human milk and the influence of procedures on immunological components of human milk. Acta Paediatr Suppl 1999;88(430): 14–8.

23. Braga LP, Palhares DB. Effect of evaporation and pasteurization in the biochemical and immunological composition of human milk. J Pediatr (Rio J) 2007;83(1): 59–63.

24. Akinbi H, Meinzen-Derr J, Auer C, et al. Alterations in the host defense properties of human milk following prolonged storage or pasteurization. J Pediatr Gastroenterol Nutr 2010;51(3):347–52.

25. Czank C, Prime DK, Hartmann B, et al. Retention of the immunological proteins of pasteurized human milk in relation to pasteurizer design and practice. Pediatr Res 2009;66(4):374–9.

26. Bertino E, Coppa GV, Giuliani F, et al. Effects of holder pasteurization on human milk oligosaccharides. Int J Immunopathol Pharmacol 2008;21(2):381–5.

27. Marx C, Bridge R, Wolf AK, et al. Human milk oligosaccharide composition differs between donor milk and mother's own milk in the NICU. J Hum Lact 2014; 30:54–61.

28. Valentine CJ, Morrow G, Fernandez S, et al. Docosahexaenoic acid and amino acid contents in pasteurized donor milk are low for preterm infants. J Pediatr 2010;157(6):906–10.

29. Vieira AA, Soares FV, Pimenta HP, et al. Analysis of the influence of pasteurization, freezing/thawing, and offer processes on human milk's macronutrient concentrations. Early Hum Dev 2011;87(8):577–80.

30. Goes HC, Torres AG, Donangelo CM, et al. Nutrient composition of banked human milk in Brazil and influence of processing on zinc distribution in milk fractions. Nutrition 2002;18(7–8):590–4.

31. Ewaschuk JB, Unger S, Harvey S, et al. Effect of pasteurization on immune components of milk: implications for feeding preterm infants. Appl Physiol Nutr Metab 2011;36(2):175–82.

32. Silvestre D, Miranda M, Muriach M, et al. Antioxidant capacity of human milk: effect of thermal conditions for the pasteurization. Acta Paediatr 2008;97(8): 1070–4.

33. Wojcik KY, Rechtman DJ, Lee ML, et al. Macronutrient analysis of a nationwide sample of donor breast milk. J Am Diet Assoc 2009;109(1):137–40.

34. Schanler RJ, Oh W. Composition of breast milk obtained from mothers of premature infants as compared to breast milk obtained from donors. J Pediatr 1980; 96(4):679–81.

35. Drulis JM, Ziegler EE. Donor human milk for premature infants, mother's milk of Iowa. Presented at the 14th ISRHML International Conference. Perth, Australia. In. Perth, Australia, January 31–February 5, 2008.
36. Lepri L, Del Bubba M, Maggini R, et al. Effect of pasteurization and storage on some components of pooled human milk. J Chromatogr B Biomed Sci Appl 1997;704(1–2):1–10.
37. Baack ML, Norris AW, Yao J, et al. Long-chain polyunsaturated fatty acid levels in US donor human milk: meeting the needs of premature infants? J Perinatol 2012;32(8):598–603.
38. Brenna JT, Varamini B, Jensen RG, et al. Docosahexaenoic and arachidonic acid concentrations in human breast milk worldwide. Am J Clin Nutr 2007; 85(6):1457–64.
39. Boyd CA, Quigley MA, Brocklehurst P. Donor breast milk versus infant formula for preterm infants: systematic review and meta-analysis. Arch Dis Child Fetal Neonatal Ed 2007;92(3):F169–75.
40. Quigley MA, Henderson G, Anthony MY, et al. Formula milk versus donor breast milk for feeding preterm or low birth weight infants. Cochrane Database Syst Rev 2007;(4):CD002971.
41. Cooper PA, Rothberg AD, Pettifor JM, et al. Growth and biochemical response of premature infants fed pooled preterm milk or special formula. J Pediatr Gastroenterol Nutr 1984;3(5):749–54.
42. Gross SJ. Growth and biochemical response of preterm infants fed human milk or modified infant formula. N Engl J Med 1983;308(5):237–41.
43. Tyson JE, Lasky RE, Mize CE, et al. Growth, metabolic response, and development in very-low-birth-weight infants fed banked human milk or enriched formula. I. Neonatal findings. J Pediatr 1983;103(1):95–104.
44. Colaizy TT, Morriss FH. Positive effect of NICU admission on breastfeeding of preterm US infants in 2000 to 2003. J Perinatol 2008;28(7):505–10.
45. Jegier BJ, Johnson TJ, Engstrom JL, et al. The institutional cost of acquiring 100 mL of human milk for very low birth weight infants in the neonatal intensive care unit. J Hum Lact 2013;29(3):390–9.
46. Sullivan S, Schanler RJ, Kim JH, et al. An exclusively human milk-based diet is associated with a lower rate of necrotizing enterocolitis than a diet of human milk and bovine milk-based products. J Pediatr 2010;156(4):562–7.e1.
47. Cristofalo EA, Schanler RJ, Blanco CL, et al. Randomized trial of exclusive human milk versus preterm formula diets in extremely premature infants. J Pediatr 2013;163(6):1592–5.e1.
48. Lucas A, Gore SM, Cole TJ, et al. Multicentre trial on feeding low birthweight infants: effects of diet on early growth. Arch Dis Child 1984;59(8):722–30.
49. O'Connor DL, Jacobs J, Hall R, et al. Growth and development of premature infants fed predominantly human milk, predominantly premature infant formula, or a combination of human milk and premature formula. J Pediatr Gastroenterol Nutr 2003;37(4):437–46.
50. Ehrenkranz RA, Dusick AM, Vohr BR, et al. Growth in the neonatal intensive care unit influences neurodevelopmental and growth outcomes of extremely low birth weight infants. Pediatrics 2006;117(4):1253–61.
51. Colaizy TT, Carlson S, Saftlas AF, et al. Growth in VLBW infants fed predominantly fortified maternal and donor human milk diets: a retrospective cohort study. BMC Pediatr 2012;12:124.
52. Hair AB, Hawthorne KM, Chetta KE, et al. Human milk feeding supports adequate growth in infants ≤ 1250 grams birth weight. BMC Res Notes 2013;6(1):459.

53. Wight NE. Donor human milk for preterm infants. J Perinatol 2001;21(4):249.

54. Anderson JW, Johnstone BM, Remley DT. Breast-feeding and cognitive development: a meta-analysis. Am J Clin Nutr 1999;70(4):525–35.

55. Weisglas-Kuperus N, Hille ET, Duivenvoorden HJ, et al. Intelligence of very preterm or very low birthweight infants in young adulthood. Arch Dis Child Fetal Neonatal Ed 2009;94(3):F196–200.

56. Lucas A, Morley R, Cole TJ, et al. A randomised multicentre study of human milk versus formula and later development in preterm infants. Arch Dis Child Fetal Neonatal Ed 1994;70(2):F141–6.

57. Section on Breastfeeding. Breastfeeding and the use of human milk. Pediatrics 2012;129(3):e827–41.

58. Arslanoglu S, Corpeleijn W, Moro G, et al. Donor human milk for preterm infants: current evidence and research directions. J Pediatr Gastroenterol Nutr 2013; 57(4):535–42.

LCPUFAs as Conditionally Essential Nutrients for Very Low Birth Weight and Low Birth Weight Infants

Metabolic, Functional, and Clinical Outcomes—How Much is Enough?

Maria Makrides, RD, PhD[a,b,*], Ricardo Uauy, MD, PhD[c]

KEYWORDS

- Preterm • Low birth weight infants • Very low birth weight infants • LCPUFA
- Randomized controlled trials • Development

KEY POINTS

- Preterm infants have a high requirement for preformed dietary docosahexaenoic acid (DHA), approximately three times the concentration in mature human milk or infant formula, if they are to meet the in utero rapid accumulation of DHA that normally occurs in late pregnancy.
- Long-chain polyunsaturated fatty acid (LCPUFA) intervention trials before 2000 mostly assessed whether infant formulas that lacked LCPUFA should be supplemented to the equivalent concentrations of DHA and other LCPUFAs typically found in human milk of women from Westernized societies.
- Trials of LCPUFA-supplemented formulas demonstrate that supplementation with at least 0.3% total fatty acids as n-3 LCPUFA improved visual development, especially in infants born less than 30-weeks gestation or with birth weights less than 1500 g.

Continued

Disclosures: M. Makrides receives honoraria (payable to her institution) for scientific advisory board contributions to Fonterra, Nestle Nutrition Institute, and Nutricia.
Associated honoraria for M. Makrides are used for professional development of students and early career researchers.
[a] Healthy Mothers, Babies and Children, South Australian Health and Medical Research Institute, North Terrace, Adelaide, South Australia, 5000, Australia; [b] Women's and Children's Health Research Institute, University of Adelaide, 72 King William Road, North Adelaide, South Australia 5006, Australia; [c] Division of Neonatology, Department of Pediatrics, Catholic University Medical School and Institute of Nutrition, INTA University of Chile, Santiago, Chile
* Corresponding author. Women's and Children's Health Research Institute, 72 King William Road, North Adelaide, South Australia 5006, Australia.
E-mail address: maria.makrides@health.sa.gov.au

http://dx.doi.org/10.1016/j.clp.2014.02.012
0095-5108/14/$ – see front matter © 2014 Elsevier Inc. All rights reserved. **perinatology.theclinics.com**

Continued

- Attention is now focused on determining whether there is added advantage to meeting the in utero accumulation rate of DHA.
- The largest intervention trial to date indicates that higher dose DHA may improve cognitive scores, reduce the risk of developmental delay, and reduce the risk of bronchopulmonary dysplasia in the smallest and most immature infants.

INTRODUCTION

In examining the effects of long-chain polyunsaturated fatty acids (LCPUFAs) on the clinical and developmental outcomes of preterm children, it is considered it logical to evaluate the early trials of formula feeding in relatively healthy low birth weight (LBW) and very low birth weight (VLBW) infants separately from the more recent controlled trials that assessed higher doses of LCPUFA. In particular, the roles of long-chain n-3 fatty acids (ie, eicosapentaenoic acid 20:5 n-3 [EPA] and docosahexaenoic acid 22:6 n-3 [DHA]) in more immature, sicker preterm infants are considered.

The early randomized controlled trials of LCPUFA interventions were designed to assess whether the infant formula for preterm infants required supplementation with n-3 and n-6 LCPUFA. At that time, formulas were devoid of all LCPUFA and contained only the precursor essential fatty acid (EFA), n-3 alpha-linolenic acid 18:3n-3 (ALA), in small amounts and much larger quantities of the n-6 EFA, linoleic acid 18:2 n-6 (LA) (**Fig. 1**).

These trials, limited to preterm infants who were exclusively fed formula from the time enteral feeding began, compared formulas containing only precursor EFAs with those supplemented with LCPUFA. Initial studies focused only on n-3 LCPUFA supplementation through fish oils. Later studies included the n-6 LCPUFA arachidonic

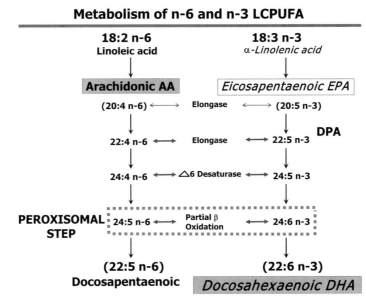

Metabolism of n-6 and n-3 LCPUFA

Fig. 1. Schema showing the metabolism of n-6 and n-3 essential fatty acids to their long chain polyunsaturated fatty acid derivatives.

acid 20:4n-6 (AA) to try to mimic the concentrations of LCPUFA in the human milk of women from Westernized societies. The infants studied were selected from those healthy enough to receive enteral feeds; few of these infants had birth weights less than 1000 g. Almost none of these intervention trials of formula feeding intervened with DHA concentrations that exceeded approximately 0.3% of total fatty acids. However, the first set of studies used deodorized menhaden oil as a source of DHA. This oil contained approximately 0.3% to 0.4% DHA but also provided approximately 0.6% EPA; therefore, the total amount of $\geq$C 20 n-3 LCPUFA was close to 1%. These early studies, which focused on the effects on biochemical endpoints and sensory or cortical neurodevelopment, were of small sample size and thus were not powered to examine relevant clinical outcomes. Collectively, these studies led to the gradual inclusion of both n-6 and n-3 LCPUFAs to premature and, later, to full term infant formula. By the year 2000, infant formula for preterm infants in developed countries was universally supplemented with LCPUFAs equivalent to the concentration found in mature human milk of women from Westernized societies. Attention since then has focused on determining the optimal dose of DHA required by preterm infants.

LCPUFA FETAL ACCRETION RATE AND METABOLISM IN PRETERM INFANTS

The measurement of fetal accretion and early ex utero accretion rates represent a relatively common approach to estimate a minimum dietary requirement. The amount of nutrient required to match accretion at the corresponding postconceptional age represents the absolute minimum for the specific nutrient required by preterm infants. In addition, this amount needs to be corrected by relative absorption of the nutrient from human milk or infant formulas and by the oxidative losses because not all that is ingested is absorbed and some of what enters the body is used as fuel and cannot be considered available for tissue deposition. Therefore, the recommendation can be derived by considering the minimum amount that needs to be taken to compensate the absorptive losses that will result in a net retention rate similar to the intrauterine accretion rate. Most attention has focused on DHA accumulation in the central nervous system. Whether the brain is preferentially protected when availability of DHA is limited is not known; however, the ease with which fetal-brain DHA is altered by maternal dietary n-3 fatty acid intake suggests that the membrane lipid composition of the fetal brain is sensitive to changes in DHA supply.[1] Because most LCPUFAs accumulate in white adipose tissue and, to a lesser extent, in lean mass and the liver,[2] it is important to consider accumulation of DHA and other LCPUFAs in all relevant organs.

Analyses of fetal autopsy tissue yield estimates of intrauterine accretion of LCPUFAs during the last trimester. These include LA, 106 mg/kg/d; ALA, 4 mg/kg/d; AA, 212 mg/kg/d; and DHA, 43 mg/kg/d.[2] It is likely that the accumulation of LCPUFAs is not linear during the last trimester. Using these numbers to calculate average daily rates of fatty acid accumulation will overestimate or underestimate tissue requirements during specific periods of growth. A more precise estimate of the fetal accretion rate cannot be determined until more data become available. However, these data based on postmortem tissue analyses of stillbirths suggest that during the third trimester in utero whole-body accumulation of DHA is of the order of 60 mg/kg/d.[2]

Based on this information, it is estimated that preterm infants who are born early and denied the rapid accumulation of DHA occurring predominantly during the last trimester of pregnancy require DHA greater than or equal to 1% total fatty acids.[3] Current research is focusing on supplementation strategies to increase the LCPUFA concentration in both human milk and infant formula from approximately 0.3% to 1% total fatty acids as DHA to match ex utero intakes with in utero accretion during the third

SINGLETON HOSPITAL
STAFF LIBRARY

trimester. This article examines the relevant trials in two sections: (1) trials related to the effects of LCPUFA supplementation of infant formula (comparing no LCPUFA vs LCPUFA equivalent with human milk levels) and (2) trials reporting the effects of LCPUFA supplementation that assessed higher doses (comparing LCPUFA concentrations equivalent with human milk vs estimated in utero accretion levels).

EFFECT OF LCPUFA SUPPLEMENTATION OF INFANT FORMULA ON VISUAL DEVELOPMENT OF PRETERM INFANTS

The role of LCPUFA, particularly that of DHA, has been a point of intense investigation since the early 1990s when the first published clinical study showed that electroretinographic function and cortical processing of visual stimuli, as measured by visual evoked potentials of preterm human infants born weighing less than 1500 g, was improved following supplementation of formula with marine oil rich in n-3 LCPUFA (0.36% of total fatty acids) compared with a control formula high in LA (n-6 EFA present in corn oil) without n-3 LCPUFA and with only trace amounts of ALA, the metabolic precursor of DHA.[4,5] A third group in the intervention study included infants who were fed formula containing soy oil as a source of ALA. The retinal and cortical function of the infants in the soy-oil formula group were intermediate between the control and marine oil group, indicating that preformed n-3 LCPUFA was needed for optimal function (matching the performance of human milk-fed neonates) (**Fig. 2**).[4,5] Importantly, the visual function of the n-3 LCPUFA–supplemented infants at 36-weeks postconceptual age did not differ from a reference group of infants fed human milk, which contains LCPUFA, or from a group of neonates born at the equivalent postconceptional age studied soon after birth.[4] The poignancy of these early observations stems from the control formula used in this clinical study. It derived most of its

Effect of early diet on Retinal function (VLBW)

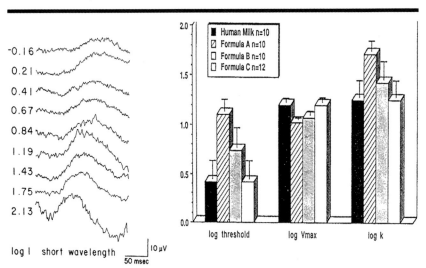

Fig. 2. Effect of early diet on retinal function of very low birth weight infants. Formula A represents a corn oil based infant formula, Formula B contained soy oil while Formula C contained a mixture of soy oil and marine oil. (*Adapted from* Uauy RD, Birch DG, Birch EE, et al. Effect of dietary omega-3 fatty acids on retinal function of very-low-birth-weight neonates. Pediatr Res 1990;28:485–92; with permission.)

PUFA from corn oil[4] and had a fatty acid composition similar to the n-3 fatty acid–deficient diet used by Neuringer and colleagues.[6,7] They showed that infant rhesus monkeys fed n-3 fatty acid–deficient formula experienced visual loss that was associated with reductions in brain DHA concentration, compared with infant monkeys fed their mothers' milk or the n-3 fatty acid–sufficient diet based on soy oil.

The follow-up assessments of this study showed similar effects on visual acuity at 4-months corrected age using electrophysiological assessments.[5] The 1990s and early 2000s saw several randomized intervention trials of formula supplemented with LCPUFA and many of these studies focused their efficacy assessment on visual function during infancy. The relevant trials are summarized in the most recent Cochrane systematic review and, although the review concludes that there is no consistent benefit of LCPUFA supplementation of infant formulas for preterm infants on visual development, it acknowledges that major differences in assessment methods between studies does not allow for a meta-analysis to be performed.[8] It is, therefore, interesting to consider the differences between the trials that did report some improvement in visual maturity with LCPUFA supplementation compared with the trials reporting no effects. It seems two factors may be influential: (1) the dose of n-3 LCPUFA or DHA supplied and (2) the maturity of the infants included in the trials. Trials of n-3 LCPUFA supplementation are more likely to report a beneficial effect on visual development if most infants included were less than 30-weeks gestation or less than 1500 g, and the dietary intervention contained at least 0.3% total fatty acids as n-3 LCPUFA.[4,9,10] Further analysis to explain the heterogeneity in responses across different studies has considered the preformed DHA consumed as well as the potential contribution to the DHA pool from the endogenous conversion of ALA to DHA. Measurements of DHA formation from deuterium-labeled ALA have revealed low levels of conversion for preterm infants (3%–5%), this is further compromised by intrauterine growth retardation.[11] Thus, only a small fraction of the ALA fed to a group of growth-retarded infants and/or LBW infants is converted to DHA. A meta-regression dose-response analysis of the effect of DHA supply on visual-acuity measures in term infants across multiple studies considered the preformed DHA consumed as well as the total DHA equivalents formed from ALA desaturation and elongation. Allowing for a potential 1%, 5%, and 10% conversion, they revealed a progressively stronger correlation reaching 0.7 when a 10% endogenous formation was from ALA.[12] A similar approach with trials involving preterm infants may be useful to better understand the difference between individual trials.

EFFECTS OF LCPUFA SUPPLEMENTATION OF INFANT FORMULA ON GLOBAL INDICES OF DEVELOPMENT

Beyond visual function,[7] different randomized trials of formula feeding with LCPUFA have assessed global indices of neurodevelopment, generally using the Bayley Scales of Infant and Toddler Development (BSITD).[10,13–18] Although some developmental scientists criticize the use of these global indices as being blunt measures of specific developmental domains, they nevertheless provide standardized measures that are useful to clinicians and families alike.

The outcomes of these[7] trials with Bayley developmental quotients (DQs) from either the first or second version of the BSITD are summarized in two relatively recent systematic reviews.[8,19] The two reviews had somewhat different approaches to combining the data in meta-analyses and, as a result, have differing outcomes. Schulzke and colleagues[8] separately reported DQs of preterm children at 12- and 18-months corrected age despite that the BSITD is age standardized. They showed no significant difference in cognitive DQ between groups at either age. Four trials included 364 preterm infants at 12-months corrected age (weighted mean difference [WMD], 0.96 points, 95% CI −1.42 to 3.34) and three trials included 494 preterm infants (WMD 2.4 points, 95% CI −0.33 to 5.12) at 18-months corrected age.[8] On the other hand, Smithers and colleagues[19] combined the 12- and 18-month data because all of the DQ scores are age standardized. They conducted a subgroup analysis according to the first BSITD version because the second version of the BSITD included more language and problem-solving items for 12- to 18-month-old children compared with the first version, as well as differences in scoring and administration. Smithers and colleagues[19] found that in the meta-analysis of all seven trials, the cognitive DQ of LCPUFA-treated preterm formula-fed children did not differ from the control in 976 preterm infants (WMD 2.13 points, 95% CI −0.87 to 5.14). However, the meta-analysis of data from the BSITD version II demonstrated an advantage of LCPUFA treatment in five trials with 879 infants (WMD, 3.4 points, 95% CI 0.56–6.31). These five trials included the most infants and were less likely than other trials to be subject to biases.

Beyond 18 months, only one published study has followed children into childhood to determine cognitive effects of LCPUFA supplementation in infancy.[20] They found no difference in intelligence quotient but did report that girls who received LCPUFA supplemented formula performed significantly better at single-word reading accuracy and spelling than girls who received unsupplemented formula.[20] However, the study was limited by large losses to follow-up (55%) making interpretation and generalization difficult. It, therefore, seems that the question of whether LCPUFA supplementation of preterm infant formula results in long-term neurodevelopmental benefit remains open and may be difficult to definitively answer because formulas for preterm infants are now all supplemented with LCPUFA.

LCPUFA NEEDS FOR LBW AND VLBW INFANTS AFFECTED BY COMMON DISEASES OF PREMATURITY

Thinking about the potential benefits of dietary LCPUFA on the diseases of prematurity demands due consideration of the importance of n-3 and n-6 LCPUFA in modulating the inflammatory immune response as well as the effects of these EFA on endothelial function, coagulation, inflammation, and neural tissue recovery after ischemic or hypoxic injury. These processes define the severity or potential recovery from hypoxic or ischemic injury.[21]

Many of the randomized controlled trials comparing the outcomes of preterm infants receiving supplemented formulas with DHA or both DHA and AA with the outcomes of infants receiving unsupplemented formula have reported a range of clinical outcomes, including necrotizing enterocolitis, sepsis, retinopathy or prematurity, intraventricular hemorrhage, and bronchopulmonary dysplasia (BPD). The relevant trials have been summarized in a systematic review and meta-analysis.[19] Because the clinical signs and symptoms used to diagnose these diseases may differ between neonatal units and may change with improvements in clinical practice over time, two sensitivity analyses were conducted. Apart from combining all data, sensitivity analyses only included trials using internationally accepted definitions of the relevant diseases or trials with a low risk of bias based on reporting adequate concealment of randomization and analysis according to the intention-to-treat principle. In meta-analyses of data from about 1500 preterm infants, the risk of necrotizing enterocolitis and sepsis did not differ between infants fed LCPUFA supplemented or control formula when all available data were included, when necrotizing enterocolitis or sepsis were confirmed according to international standards or in the trial quality sensitivity analysis.[19] In overall analyses, there were no clear differences in retinopathy of prematurity, intraventricular hemorrhage, or BPD between preterm infants fed LCPUFA-supplemented or control formula. There were also no differences when trials reported diseases according to the prespecified definitions or in the quality of trial sensitivity analysis. However, the data were limited by small sample sizes and potential biases associated with the studies and the definitions of the diseases.[19]

EFFECTS OF LCPUFA SUPPLEMENTATION DESIGNED TO MIMIC IN UTERO ACCUMULATION

With the publication of two relevant intervention trials in the last 5 years,[22,23] attention has turned to whether dietary DHA supplementation to match in utero supply results in measurable benefits to the growth, development, or clinical outcomes of children born preterm. One trial focused on human milk–fed preterm infants,[22] whereas the other was inclusive of all infants regardless of whether they were fed human milk, formula, or a mixture.[23] Henriksen and colleagues[22] randomly allocated 141 VLBW infants (<1500 g) who were human milk fed to 32 mg of DHA and 31 mg of AA per 100 mL milk and demonstrated an improvement in problem-solving at 6-months corrected age. In a follow-up at 20 months of age, they showed no difference in cognitive DQ but there was a significant improvement in sustained attention in free-play activities.[24] No other differences in clinical outcomes were reported.[22,24] The relatively small sample size and losses to follow-up make interpretation difficult.

The single largest trial, involving more than 650 infants born less than 33 weeks, was designed to assess the delivery of approximately 1% total fatty acids with DHA compared with approximately 0.3% DHA supplied either through human milk, infant formula, or a combination to mimic typical feeding practices in neonatal units.[23] All milks contained 0.4% to 0.5% total fatty acids as AA. The trial was powered for neurodevelopmental outcomes and reported on outcomes related to visual development, growth, and the typical diseases of prematurity. Although there were no significant differences between groups in overall cognitive DQ at 18-months corrected age (WMD 1.9; 95% CI -1.0 to 4.7), severe cognitive delay (score <70) was reduced from 10.5% in the control group to 5% in the higher DHA group (relative risk 0.50; 95% CI 0.26–0.93).[23] Furthermore, there were significant treatment interactions indicating that higher DHA treatment had differential responses by infant sex and birth weight category. Girls had a significant improvement in cognitive DQ with high-DHA treatment, whereas boys did not differ between groups. For infants born weighing less than 1250 g, the cognitive DQ in the high-DHA group was higher than with standard DHA and there were no group difference in infants born weighing at least 1250 g (**Fig. 3**).

In secondary analyses relating to the clinical outcomes of infants, there were no group differences relating to the incidence of sepsis, necrotizing enterocolitis, or intraventricular hemorrhage; however, high-DHA treatment may result in lower rates of BPD, particularly in infants born weighing less than 1250 g and male infants.[23,25] Other secondary analyses indicated that the high-DHA group had better visual acuity at 4 months of age compared with the standard-DHA group[26] and that infants fed higher DHA were 0.7 cm longer at 18-months corrected age (95% CI 0.1–1.4, $P = .02$).[27] There was an interaction effect between treatment and birth weight strata for weight and length. Higher DHA resulted in increased length in infants born weighing less than or equal to 1250 g, at 4-months corrected age, and in weight and length at 12- and 18-months corrected age.[27] Although complex, these data indicate that

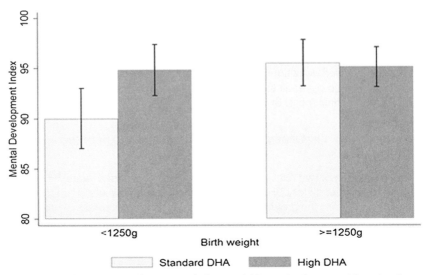

Fig. 3. Effect of high DHA (~1% total fatty acids) on Bayley cognitive development compared with standard DHA (~0.3% total fatty acids as DHA) by birth weight strata. (*Adapted from* Makrides M, Gibson RA, McPhee AJ, et al. Neurodevelopmental outcomes of preterm infants fed high-dose docosahexaenoic acid: a randomized controlled trial. JAMA 2009;301:175–82.)

DHA up to 1% total dietary fatty acids is safe, does not adversely affect growth, and may have other clinical advantages in relation to BPD and early childhood neurodevelopmental outcomes for important subgroups of infants. The relatively consistent benefit of higher dietary DHA, designed to emulate in utero accretion, in the smallest and most immature infants is consistent with the hypothesis that suboptimal DHA availability during the critical neonatal period results in disturbed DHA accumulation has consequences on development. Current large-scale trials, such as N3RO (N-3 LCPUFA for Respiratory Outcomes in Infants Born <29 weeks), should provide conclusive and contemporary data for higher dose DHA supplementation to the most vulnerable infants as well as offer some new insights into the mechanisms by which higher dose dietary DHA may work to dampen inflammatory immune responses.

FUTURE DIRECTIONS OF RELEVANCE TO NEONATAL AND PERINATAL MEDICINE

Over the past three decades, knowledge of DHA effects on gene expression and on the production of n-3–derived eicosanoids has expanded significantly beyond the areas covered in this short review. Animal studies using a genetic modification have produced a rat that overexpresses delta-6 desaturase (fat-1 rat), allowing significant experimentation in animals that have increased DHA content of all tissues. In addition, studies can be done on unique models of stroke as a hypoxic injury that can be treated with DHA-derived compounds capable of resolving the associated inflammatory insult. Owing to their potential relevance to neonatal health and/or amelioration of neonatal conditions affecting VLBW infants, the authors suggest some areas in which further research may reveal significant benefits:

1. Prevention of excessive inflammation, especially in the gut and lung, and understanding of some of the mechanisms by which dietary n-3 LCPUFA may alter the onset and progression of necrotizing enterocolitis and BPD.

2. Protection from hypoxic or ischemic organ damage as demonstrated by the use of DHA derivatives in ischemic brain infarctions and may have relevance to the hypoxic or ischemic brain injury experienced with intraventricular hemorrhage.
3. Some of the latest trials suggesting that higher dose DHA administered in pregnancy reduces the risk of early preterm birth may offer additional treatment modalities with potential to administer DHA to mothers who potentially will deliver preterm or growth-retarded infants to prevent or ameliorate the later consequences of these conditions.

SUMMARY

The essentiality of LCPUFA, particularly DHA, for preterm infants has been a point of discussion in the literature for some 25 years. Although most of the biochemical studies clearly show the insufficiency of DHA in the diet of preterm infants, the picture has not been so clear from the intervention trials with clinical and developmental outcomes. The early intervention trials, and most of the controlled trials, were designed to assess whether infant formulas that were devoid of LCPUFA should be supplemented to the equivalent concentrations of DHA and other LCPUFA found in typical human milk. Intervention studies involving exclusively formula-fed preterm infants have demonstrated improved visual development using neurosensory and behavioral techniques. The trials showing the most consistent benefit included those in which most infants were born less than 30-weeks gestation or had birth weights less than 1500 g and the dietary intervention contained at least 0.3% total fatty acids as n-3 LCPUFA. With the universal supplementation of all preterm infant formula with LCPUFA since the year 2000, attention has focused on determining the specific dietary requirement of DHA and whether there is added advantage to meeting the in utero accumulation rate of DHA, which is approximately three times the concentration in most human milk and infant formula.

To date, the largest intervention trial addressing this question indicates that higher dose DHA may improve cognitive scores, reduce the risk of developmental delay, and reduce the risk of bronchopulmonary dysplasia in the smallest and most immature infants.

REFERENCES

1. Innis SM. Essential fatty acid transfer and fetal development. Placenta 2005; 26(Suppl A):S70–5.
2. Lapillonne A, Jensen CL. Reevaluation of the DHA requirement for the premature infant. Prostaglandins Leukot Essent Fatty Acids 2009;81:143–50.
3. Lapillonne A, Groh-Wargo S, Gonzalez CH, et al. Lipid needs of preterm infants: updated recommendations. J Pediatr 2013;162:S37–47.
4. Uauy RD, Birch DG, Birch EE, et al. Effect of dietary omega-3 fatty acids on retinal function of very-low-birth-weight neonates. Pediatr Res 1990;28:485–92.
5. Birch EE, Birch DG, Hoffman DR, et al. Dietary essential fatty acid supply and visual acuity development. Invest Ophthalmol Vis Sci 1992;33:3242–53.
6. Neuringer M, Connor WE, Lin DS, et al. Biochemical and functional effects of prenatal and postnatal omega 3 fatty acid deficiency on retina and brain in rhesus monkeys. Proc Natl Acad Sci U S A 1986;83:4021–5.
7. Neuringer M, Connor WE, Van Petten C, et al. Dietary omega-3 fatty acid deficiency and visual loss in infant rhesus monkeys. J Clin Invest 1984;73:272–6.
8. Schulzke SM, Patole SK, Simmer K. Long-chain polyunsaturated fatty acid supplementation in preterm infants. Cochrane Database Syst Rev 2011;(2):CD000375.

9. Carlson SE, Werkman SH, Rhodes PG, et al. Visual-acuity development in healthy preterm infants: effect of marine-oil supplementation. Am J Clin Nutr 1993;58:35–42.

10. O'Connor DL, Hall R, Adamkin D, et al. Growth and development in preterm infants fed long-chain polyunsaturated fatty acids: a prospective, randomized controlled trial. Pediatrics 2001;108:359–71.

11. Llanos A, Lin Y, Mena P, et al. Infants with intrauterine growth restriction have impaired formation of docosahexaenoic acid in early neonatal life: a stable isotope study. Pediatr Res 2005;58:735–40.

12. Uauy R, Hoffman DR, Mena P, et al. Term infant studies of DHA and ARA supplementation on neurodevelopment: results of randomized controlled trials. J Pediatr 2003;143:S17–25.

13. van Wezel-Meijler G, van der Knaap MS, Huisman J, et al. Dietary supplementation of long-chain polyunsaturated fatty acids in preterm infants: effects on cerebral maturation. Acta Paediatr 2002;91:942–50.

14. Fewtrell MS, Morley R, Abbott RA, et al. Double-blind, randomized trial of long-chain polyunsaturated fatty acid supplementation in formula fed to preterm infants. Pediatrics 2002;110:73–82.

15. Fewtrell MS, Abbott RA, Kennedy K, et al. Randomized, double-blind trial of long-chain polyunsaturated fatty acid supplementation with fish oil and borage oil in preterm infants. J Pediatr 2004;144:471–9.

16. Clandinin MT, Van Aerde JE, Merkel KL, et al. Growth and development of preterm infants fed infant formulas containing docosahexaenoic acid and arachidonic acid. J Pediatr 2005;146:461–8.

17. Fang PC, Kuo HK, Huang CB, et al. The effect of supplementation of docosahexaenoic acid and arachidonic acid on visual acuity and neurodevelopment in larger preterm infants. Chang Gung Med J 2005;28:708–15.

18. Carlson SE, Cooke RJ, Werkman SH, et al. First year growth of preterm infants fed standard compared to marine oil n-3 supplemented formula. Lipids 1992;27:901–7.

19. Smithers LG, Gibson RA, McPhee AJ, et al. Effect of LCPUFA supplementation of preterm infants on disease risk and neurodevelopment: a systematic review of randomised controlled trials. Am J Clin Nutr 2008;87:912–20.

20. Isaacs EB, Ross S, Kennedy K, et al. 10-year cognition in preterms after random assignment to fatty acid supplementation in infancy. Pediatrics 2011;128:e890–8.

21. Bazan NG, Molina MF, Gordon WC. Docosahexaenoic acid signalolipidomics in nutrition: significance in aging, neuroinflammation, macular degeneration, Alzheimer's, and other neurodegenerative diseases. Annu Rev Nutr 2011;31:321–51.

22. Henriksen C, Haugholt K, Lindgren M, et al. Improved cognitive development among preterm infants attributable to early supplementation of human milk with docosahexaenoic acid and arachidonic acid. Pediatrics 2008;121:1137–45.

23. Makrides M, Gibson RA, McPhee AJ, et al. Neurodevelopmental outcomes of preterm infants fed high-dose docosahexaenoic acid: a randomized controlled trial. JAMA 2009;301:175–82.

24. Westerberg AC, Schei R, Henriksen C, et al. Attention among very low birth weight infants following early supplementation with docosahexaenoic and arachidonic acid. Acta Paediatr 2011;100:47–52.

25. Manley BJ, Makrides M, Collins CT, et al. High-dose docosahexaenoic acid supplementation of preterm infants: respiratory and allergy outcomes. Pediatrics 2011;128:e71–7.

26. Smithers LG, Gibson RA, McPhee A, et al. Higher dose of docosahexaenoic acid in the neonatal period improves visual acuity of preterm infants: results of a randomized controlled trial. Am J Clin Nutr 2008;88:1049–56.
27. Collins CT, Makrides M, Gibson RA, et al. Pre- and post-term growth in pre-term infants supplemented with higher-dose DHA: a randomised controlled trial. Br J Nutr 2011;105(11):1635–43.

Post-discharge Nutrition and the VLBW Infant: To Supplement or Not Supplement?
A Review of the Current Evidence

Nneka I. Nzegwu, DO*, Richard A. Ehrenkranz, MD

KEYWORDS

- Post-discharge nutrition • Post-discharge formula • Nutrient-enriched formula
- Human milk • Multinutrient fortification • Postnatal growth failure

KEY POINTS

- Suboptimal and varied nutritional practices regarding very-low-birth-weight infants (VLBWs) in the neonatal intensive care unit contribute to continued growth failure and restriction in the post-discharge period.
- Human milk has many benefits; it is recommended solely for term infants and is the preferred source of enteral nutrition for preterm infants.
- Systematic reviews have shown limited benefits in growth and neurodevelopmental outcomes with the use of post-discharge formulas or multinutrient fortification of human milk.
- It is important to have an individualized approach to post-discharge nutrition as VLBW infants have varying rates of postnatal growth failure and restriction.

INTRODUCTION

Because of advancements in neonatology, the survival of very-low-birth-weight (VLBW; birth weight [BW] <1500 g) and extremely low-birth-weight (ELBW; BW <1000 g) infants has increased over the past several decades. Unfortunately, survival of these infants has been associated with a persistent occurrence of neonatal morbidities, such as growth failure, bronchopulmonary dysplasia (BPD), necrotizing enterocolitis (NEC), retinopathy of prematurity, late-onset infections, cerebral palsy, and neurodevelopmental impairment. Current consensus nutritional recommendations are "designed to provide nutrients to approximate the rate of growth and composition of weight gain for a normal fetus of the same postmenstrual age (PMA)".[1,2] Despite these recommendations, endorsed by the American Academy of Pediatrics (AAP) Committee on Nutrition, and other national and international organizations

Section of Neonatal-Perinatal Medicine, Department of Pediatrics, Yale University School of Medicine, 333 Cedar Street, PO Box 208064, New Haven, CT 06520-8064, USA
* Corresponding author.
E-mail address: nneka.nzegwu@yale.edu

Clin Perinatol 41 (2014) 463–474
http://dx.doi.org/10.1016/j.clp.2014.02.008   perinatology.theclinics.com
0095-5108/14/$ – see front matter © 2014 Elsevier Inc. All rights reserved.

(ESPGHAN, Life Sciences), neonatologists struggle daily to meet this goal, and post-natal growth failure and restriction are common.[3,4]

Suboptimal nutritional practices of VLBWs have been shown to contribute to a period of inadequate nutrition and poor growth.[5] Data from the National Institute for Child and Human Development Neonatal Research Network, collected from live births between 1995 and 1996, demonstrated that 97% of the VLBW population experienced growth failure with weights less than the 10th percentile at 36 weeks' PMA, and that 99% of ELBW infants were less than the 10th percentile at 36 weeks' PMA.[6] At 18 months' corrected age (CA), Dusick and colleagues[7] reported that 40% of the infants in the 501 to 1000 g BW group still had weights, lengths, and head circumferences less than the 10th percentile. Postnatal growth failure and inadequate nutrition have been associated with poor long-term neurodevelopmental outcomes. Ehrenkranz and colleagues[8] reported that more rapid in-hospital growth velocity was associated with better neurodevelopmental and growth outcomes at 18 to 22 months' CA.

Significant focus has been placed on alleviating the protein and energy deficits in the initial postnatal period, including early initiation of total parenteral nutrition (ie, amino acid proteins), use of higher protein preterm formulas, and feeding guidelines with a focus on early initiation of minimal enteral feedings.[9] Despite strides made to match intrauterine growth rates in the immediate postnatal period and during neonatal intensive care unit (NICU) hospitalization, many preterm infants continue to have growth restriction at discharge.[7,10] Furthermore, preterm infants are frequently discharged home before term equivalent age (40 weeks' CA) and less than term equivalent size. Previous studies[11–13] have shown that there may be a window for catch-up growth in the initial post-discharge period. This article reviews post-discharge nutrition in the VLBW population, examines different types of post-discharge nutrition, the current evidence, and future and remaining questions. Also provided are recommendations for post-discharge nutrition in this vulnerable population.

NUTRIENT NEEDS OF VLBW INFANTS VERSUS TERM INFANTS

Preterm infants have increased macronutrient and micronutrient requirements compared with term infants. Most of these macronutrients and micronutrients would have been acquired during the third trimester of pregnancy.[14–16] The main macronutrients (protein, fat, and carbohydrate) and micronutrients (vitamins, minerals, electrolytes, and trace elements) are needed in increased quantities to sustain rapid growth of preterm infants.[16] It is widely thought that these infants will require protein intakes of 3.5 to 4.0 g/kg/d once the continuous supply of amino acids, glucose, and essential fatty acids from the placenta ceases.[17,18] In order for bone mineralization to occur normally, VLBW infants must receive adequate intakes of protein and energy. Furthermore, during the post-discharge period, these infants continue to have greater nutritional requirements for calcium, phosphorus, and other vitamins and trace minerals (**Table 1**).[1,2]

The AAP recommends human milk as the sole nutrient for healthy, term infants for the first 6 months of life, breast-feeding to 12 months of life, and human milk as the preferred source of enteral nutrition for preterm infants.[1,19] Atkinson[20] and others have reported on the differences between the composition of term human milk and preterm human milk, especially during the early lactation period (colostrum, transitional milk). Both preterm and term human milk are inadequate in meeting the nutritional requirements of VLBW infants. Just as protein and energy are important for linear growth, micronutrients such as calcium, phosphorus, and Vitamin D are equally

Table 1
Recommended macronutrient/micronutrient requirements (units/kg/d) for the stable preterm infant

	Term	ELBW	VLBW	VLBW Postterm
Energy, kcal	90–120	130–150	110–130	90–100
Protein, g	1.52	3.8–4.4	3.4–4.2	2.0
Carbohydrate, g	16–20[a]	9–20	7–17	6.8–14.1
Fat, g	8–10.3[a]	6.2–8.4	5.3–7.2	4.0–6.6
Vitamin A, IU	1333	700–1500	700–1500	545–1273
Vitamin D, IU	200	150–400	150–400	400
Calcium, mg	70–120	100–220	100–220	253–377
Phosphorus, mg	35–75	60–140	60–140	105–273
Iron, mg	0.09[a]	2–4	2–4	1.8–2.7
Zinc, µg	666[a]	1000–3000	1000–3000	890

[a] For an average term infant 0–6 months of age.
Data from Refs.[2,18,24,29,38–40]

important in growth and bone mineralization. The AAP Committee on Nutrition recommends 150 to 220 mg/kg/d of calcium, 75 to 140 mg/kg/d of phosphorus, and 200 to 400 IU/d of vitamin D for enterally fed VLBW infants.[21] During hospitalization, human milk fortifiers added to human milk, or high protein preterm formulas, are used to meet these increased demands.

Post-discharge nutrition is an area garnering more attention, because it has been shown that preterm and extremely preterm infants are at a higher risk for growth failure at discharge and that poor growth is associated with impaired neurodevelopmental outcomes.[22,23] Currently, there are no widely accepted feeding recommendations for the post-discharge nutrition of preterm infants and no studies have elucidated any lasting effects on growth and neurodevelopmental outcomes. Post-discharge nutritional practices vary widely by NICU, individual health care providers, and country.[24] The spectrum of post-discharge nutritional practices involves a range of breast-feeding and nutrient enrichment of enteral feedings. Preterm and extremely preterm infants may vary in the extent of their growth failure and thus have the potential to be discharged home with different nutritional expectations.

Post-discharge nutrition should be thought of for 3 groups of infants: (1) the exclusively breast-fed preterm infant, (2) the breast-fed preterm infant supplemented with post-discharge formula, and (3) the preterm infant receiving post-discharge and/or term formula.

TYPES OF POST-DISCHARGE NUTRITION

Table 2 compares the composition of mature human milk with the most commonly used post-discharge and term formulas. In the hospital setting, commercially available preterm infant formulas and human milk multinutrient fortifiers have been made to address specifically the increased nutritional needs of preterm and extremely preterm infants. Multinutrient fortifiers and preterm formulas are not generally commercially available because of concerns for toxicity if the recommended intake of certain nutrients is exceeded. Preterm formulas (24 kcal/oz) have higher amounts of protein, energy, calcium, phosphorus, and other trace elements and vitamins when compared with term formulas. Post-discharge formulas are an intermediate or transitional formula between preterm and term formula with more energy (22 kcal/oz), protein

Table 2
Composition of post-discharge formulas (per 100 mL) and mature human milk

	Mature Human Milk[39]	Similac Neosure 22 kcal/oz[a]	Enfamil Enfacare 22 kcal/oz[b]	Similac Advance 20 kcal/oz[a]	Enfamil Lipil 20 kcal/oz[b]	Nestlé Good Start 20 kcal/oz[c]
Energy, kcal	65–70	74.4	74	67.6	68	67
Protein, g	1.03	2.1	2.1	1.4	1.4	1.5
Carbohydrate, g	6.7–7.0	7.5	7.9	7.2	7.4	7.5
Fat, g	3.5	4.1	3.9	3.8	3.6	3.4
Calcium, mg	20–25	78.1	89	52.8	53	44.9
Phosphorus, mg	12–14	46.1	49	28.4	29	25.5
Sodium, mg	12–25	24.5	26	16.2	18.4	18.4
Iron, mg	0.3–0.9	1.34	1.3	1.2	1.2	1.0

[a] Mead Johnson Nutritionals, Evansville, IN; http://www.meadjohnson.com/Brands/Pages/Products-by Need.aspx.
[b] Abbott Nutrition, Abbott Laboratories, Columbus, OH; http://abbottnutrition.com/.
[c] Gerber (Nestlé) Infant Formulas, Glendale, CA; http://medical.gerber.com/products/Default.aspx.

(2.8 g/100 kcal), calcium, phosphorus, and zinc.[25] These increased nutrient components help to promote linear growth and improve neurodevelopmental outcomes.

Feeding human milk during the NICU hospitalization has some advantages for preterm infants, such as decreased risk of NEC and sepsis, better gastrointestinal tolerance,[26] and improved neurologic outcomes at 18 months' CA and at 7 to 8 years of age.[27,28] Use of human milk fortifiers during the NICU hospitalization addresses a main disadvantage of human milk: that it does not meet the nutritional requirements for VLBW infants for protein, energy, calcium, phosphorus, and important trace elements and vitamins.[2,29] This use of human milk fortifiers raises questions regarding how to supplement human milk to provide additional nutrients if the infant is solely breast-feeding post-discharge. Specifically, what would be the most appropriate caloric density of the supplement or the amount of multinutrients that should be provided, how long should the supplementation be provided, and if supplementation in the post-discharge period leads to improved growth and neurodevelopmental outcomes.

MONITORING GROWTH IN THE POST-DISCHARGE PERIOD

Monitoring the nutritional status of preterm and extremely preterm infants is of the utmost importance as an infant nears discharge. Nutritional needs and a feeding plan should be discussed with families of preterm infants to ensure that parents understand the nutritional goals before discharge. Infants should be transitioned to the feedings they will be on at home several days to a week before discharge to ensure that the feedings are well tolerated and that the infant is taking adequate volumes and demonstrating growth. Furthermore, preterm infants should be seen by a pediatrician within 48 hours of discharge to complete an overall assessment of nutritional status. The in-hospital health care team should discuss concerns about growth and the nutritional plan as part of discharge planning to ensure a smooth transition to the outpatient care setting.[25]

Trained personnel should obtain serial measurements of weight, length, and head circumference plotted on validated growth charts to monitor postnatal growth and identify potential growth or developmental issues.[24] Two recently described growth charts, Fenton and Olsen (**Figs. 1** and **2**), can be used to follow growth in the

A **B**

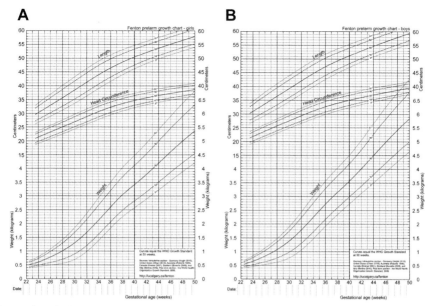

Fig. 1. (*A, B*) The Fenton preterm infant growth charts can be used to monitor postnatal growth of preterm infants from 22 weeks' gestational age to 10 weeks postterm. (*From* Fenton TR, Kim JH. A systematic review and meta-analysis to revise the Fenton growth chart for preterm infants. BMC Pediatr 2013;13:59. © 2013 Fenton and Kim. Accessed November 6, 2013.)

NICU[30] and then in the outpatient setting until 50 weeks' PMA. After 50 weeks' PMA, the Centers for Disease Control and Prevention (CDC), in conjunction with the AAP, recommend the use of the World Health Organization (WHO) growth charts[19] until 24 months' CA to monitor growth. The Fenton growth chart[31] is gender-specific and based on a meta-analysis of 6 population-based reports. The Olsen intrauterine growth curves[32] are derived from an administrative data set from the Pediatrix Medical Group based on a large, diverse sample consisting of 257,855 US infants between 23 and 41 weeks' gestation. Growth and nutritional assessments should be obtained every 2 to 4 weeks in the early post-discharge period until stable weight gain is established.

Preterm infants who are predominantly breast-fed, or who have significant morbidities such as BPD, should be monitored very closely in the outpatient setting. Pediatricians should advocate and provide support for the establishment and continuation of successful breast-feeding in preterm infants and coordinate additional resources, such as certified lactation consultants and nutritionists. When there is faltering growth or a decrease in growth percentiles, further investigation is warranted to determine the underlying cause. Beyond obtaining a thorough maternal and postnatal history and following up on the state newborn screening results, there are several biomarkers of nutritional status that may help in assessing for nutritional deficiencies. Hall[33] recommended an initial assessment of prealbumin, ferritin, blood urea nitrogen, and alkaline phosphatase. Because of the differing nutritional needs of preterm infants, it is important to have an individualized approach to their nutrition.

CURRENT EVIDENCE ABOUT POST-DISCHARGE NUTRITION

Because of the increasing belief that post-discharge nutrition plays a role in optimizing growth and improving long-term growth and neurodevelopmental outcomes, many

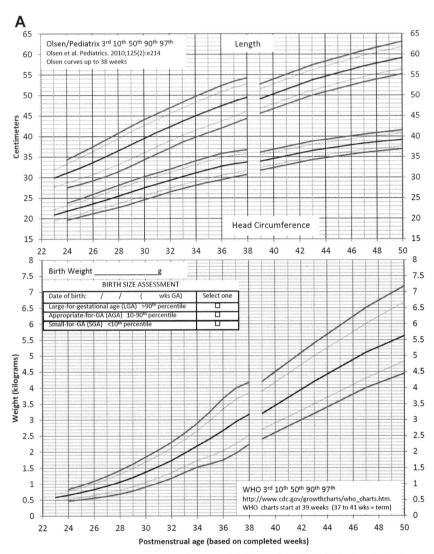

Fig. 2. (*A*) The Olsen intrauterine growth curves (girls) combined with the WHO-CDC growth charts can be used to monitor postnatal growth of preterm infants from 23 to 50 weeks' gestational age. (*B*) The Olsen intrauterine growth curves (boys) combined with the WHO-CDC growth charts can be used to monitor postnatal growth of preterm infants from 23 to 50 weeks' gestational age. (*From* Pediatrix Medical Group. Available at: http://www.pediatrix.com/workfiles/NICUGrowthCurves7.30.pdf; with permission. Accessed November 6, 2013.)

studies over the last 2 decades have examined different types of post-discharge nutrition for varying lengths of time in the preterm infant. Recent *Cochrane Reviews* have included mainly randomized controlled trials comparing nutrient-enriched formula (post-discharge formula or preterm formula) and standard term formula for preterm infants following discharge[34] and multinutrient fortification of human breast milk for preterm infants following hospital discharge.[35]

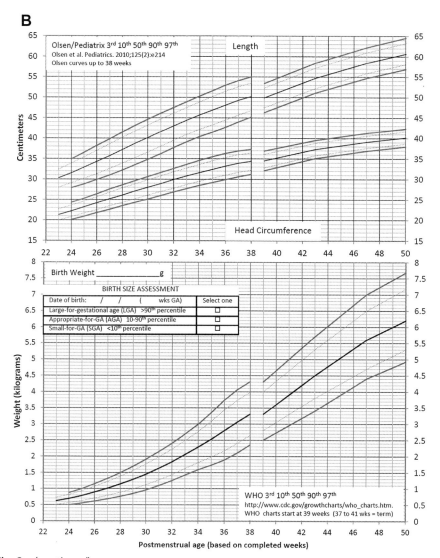

Fig. 2. (*continued*)

The first review (**Table 3**) included 15 eligible trials with 1128 preterm infants. The trials were subdivided into 2 groups: post-discharge formula versus term formula and preterm formula versus term formula. This meta-analysis did not identify a significant growth benefit associated with the use of post-discharge formulas compared with term formulas. Therefore, the results of this review do not support current expert opinion or consensus guidelines that recommend that formula-fed preterm infants should receive a post-discharge formula for up to 12 months post-discharge.[34] However, when an in-hospital preterm formula was compared with term formula post-discharge, significant increases in anthropometric indices were identified up to 12 to 18 months' CA. A limitation of these trials was that the preterm infants included were fed ad libitum and more information is needed on infants with morbidities such

Table 3
Cochrane Review: nutrient-enriched formula versus standard term formula

Post-discharge Formula vs Standard Term Formula

Anthropometrics	No. of Studies	No. of Participants	Effect Size MD	95% CI
Weight (g)				
3–4 mo CA	5	408	−3.76	[−156.67, 149.15]
6 mo CA	6	461	56.23	[−111.53, 223.98]
9 mo CA	4	347	244.09	[16.95, 471.23]
12 mo CA	2	120	71.53	[−344.06, 487.12]
18 mo CA	1	192	100.0	[−246.90, 446.90]
Crown heel length (mm)				
3–4 mo CA	5	408	4.18	[−0.77, 9.13]
6 mo CA	6	461	3.46	[−1.21, 8.13]
9 mo CA	4	347	7.33	[1.80, 12.87]
12 mo CA	2	120	−0.83	[−9.00, 9.34]
18 mo CA	1	192	9.0	[0.32, 17.68]
Head circumference (cm)				
3–4 mo CA	5	408	−0.87	[−3.73, 1.99]
6 mo CA	6	461	0.72	[−2.12, 3.56]
9 mo CA	4	347	0.16	[−3.21, 3.53]
12 mo CA	2	120	0.25	[−5.50, 6.01]
18 mo CA	1	192	−3.0	[−8.24, 2.24]
Development at 18 mo CA				
Bayley-II: MDI	1	184	0.90	[−3.24, 5.04]
Bayley-II: PDI	1	184	2.70	[−1.28, 6.68]

Preterm Formula vs Standard Term Formula

Anthropometrics	No. of Studies	No. of Participants	Effect Size MD	95% CI
Weight (g)				
3–4 mo CA	3	130	74.41	[−267.10, 415.93]
6 mo CA	4	273	74.60	[−164.73, 313.92]
9 mo CA	1	59	112.0	[−482.69, 706.69]
12 mo CA	4	265	539.48	[−255.03, 823.92]
18 mo CA	2	162	490.81	[142.19, 839.44]
Crown heel length (mm)				
3–4 mo CA	3	130	−2.27	[−13.09, 8.56]
6 mo CA	3	160	1.83	[−6.25, 9.92]
9 mo CA	1	59	−3.0	[−17.03, 11.03]
12 mo CA	3	152	5.13	[−4.23, 14.49]
18 mo CA	2	162	11.0	[1.89, 20.11]

(continued on next page)

Table 3
(continued)

| Preterm Formula vs Standard Term Formula | | | | |
| | | | Effect Size | |
Anthropometrics	No. of Studies	No. of Participants	MD	95% CI
Head circumference (mm)				
3–4 mo CA	3	130	3.61	[−2.09, 9.31]
6 mo CA	3	160	5.82	[1.32, 10.32]
9 mo CA	1	59	8.0	[0.85, 15.15]
12 mo CA	3	152	6.07	[1.07, 11.06]
18 mo CA	2	162	5.42	[0.69, 10.14]
Development at 18 mo CA				
Bayley-II: MDI	2	143	−1.44	[−6.22, 3.35]
Bayley-II: PDI	2	143	−1.13	[−4.19, 1.93]

Statistical method: mean difference (IV, Fixed, 95% CI).

Abbreviations: Bayley-II: MDI, Bayley Scales of Infant Development-II: Mental Developmental Index; Bayley-II: PDI, Bayley Scales of Infant Development-II: Psychomotor Developmental Index; CI, confidence intervals; MD, mean difference.

Data from Young L, Morgan J, McCormick FM, et al. Nutrient-enriched formula versus standard term formula for preterm infants following hospital discharge. Cochrane Database Syst Rev 2012;(3):CD004696.

as BPD and congenital heart disease because they do not feed ad libitum. None of the studies included in this review assessed the long-term growth and neurodevelopmental outcomes beyond 12 to 18 months' CA and some of the studies only have reported growth outcomes up to 6 months' CA.

In the second review,[35] 2 trials including 246 infants were identified (**Table 4**). This systematic review reported no statistically significant difference in growth rates between preterm infants fed human milk fortified with multinutrients compared with infants fed unfortified human milk post-discharge. Both studies showed that fortification

Table 4
Cochrane Review: multinutrient fortification versus no fortification of human milk

| | | | Effect Size | |
Anthropometrics	No. of Studies	No. of Participants	MD	95% CI
Weight (g)				
3–4 mo CA	2	236	138.26	[−89.87, 366.40]
12 mo CA	2	211	255.25	[−93.40, 603.90]
Length (cm)				
3–4 mo CA	2	236	0.60	[−0.14, 1.33]
12 mo CA	2	211	0.88	[0.01, 1.74]
Head circumference (cm)				
3–4 mo CA	2	235	0.22	[−0.15, 0.58]
12 mo CA	2	197	0.16	[−0.27, 0.60]

Statistical method: mean difference (IV, fixed, 95% CI).

Abbreviations: CI, confidence intervals; MD, mean difference.

Data from Young L, Embleton ND, McCormick FM, et al. Multinutrient fortification of human breast milk for preterm infants following hospital discharge. Cochrane Database Syst Rev 2013;(2):CD004866.

of human milk did not adversely affect the duration or exclusivity of breast-feeding. No data on long-term growth or neurodevelopmental outcomes beyond 18 months' CA were reported. O'Connor and colleagues[36] demonstrated no statistically significant differences for preterm infants on the Bayley II Scales for Infant Development Mental and Psychomotor Developmental Index scores at 18 months' CA. However, in a later report,[37] the investigators showed that, in the same cohort of preterm infants, those infants fed mostly a human milk diet with the addition of a multinutrient fortifier had higher grating acuity and contrast sensitivity (used a surrogate marker of neurodevelopment) than infants feed with human milk alone at 4 and 6 months' CA.

These reports suggest that the provision of post-discharge formulas or multinutrient fortification of human milk results in minimal improvements in growth and neurodevelopmental outcomes. There is currently no consistent, convincing evidence that the use of different types of post-discharge nutrition leads to significant improvements in neurodevelopmental outcomes or is more effective in supporting post-discharge growth. Further studies are needed examining long-term growth and neurodevelopmental outcomes in early childhood and adolescence and its effects (**Box 1**).

Box 1
Recommendations for post-discharge nutrition of the VLBW infant

- Post-discharge nutrition needs may be met by human milk, human milk supplemented with post-discharge or term formula, or exclusively post-discharge or term formula because systematic reviews have shown minimal benefit in growth and neurologic outcomes

- An individualized approach is essential for the post-discharge nutrition of the VLBW infant

- Human milk is preferred for preterm infants and breast-feeding should be advocated by pediatricians and lactation resources should be made available

- Before going home, a discharge nutrition plan should be discussed among the health care team, parents, and, if possible, the outpatient care provider

- Close monitoring of growth parameters using validated growth curves (weight-, length-, head circumference-for-age) and nutritional intake should be assessed at discharge and every 2 to 4 weeks thereafter, until stable weight gain is established

---

SUMMARY

There is good evidence in the literature to suggest that, despite intensive nutritional practices to improve nutrition after birth,[14] preterm and extremely preterm infants are still at a significant risk for growth failure in the immediate post-discharge period. Past studies have suggested that there may be a window of catch-up growth in which linear growth and neurodevelopmental outcomes can be affected. Optimization of in-hospital nutrition with early parenteral nutrition and early initiation of minimal enteral feedings will significantly impact the growth deficits that exist soon after birth.[9]

In addition, developing a strategy to monitor the growth and development of these preterm infants post-discharge is crucial to decreasing the risk of continued growth failure. This strategy should be individualized to each VLBW infant as nutritional needs may be wide ranging. In addition, as endorsed by the AAP and WHO, finding ways to support breast-feeding and lactation practices will serve to increase the number of preterm infants receiving breast milk or being breast-fed post-discharge, which has previously been shown to be beneficial for growth and neurodevelopmental outcomes. Further research is needed to determine if there are any growth or neurodevelopmental outcome benefits for VLBW infants beyond 18 to 24 months' CA if an individualized approach is undertaken towards post-discharge nutrition.

REFERENCES

1. American Academy of Pediatrics Committee on Nutrition. Chapter 5: nutritional needs of the preterm infant. In: Kleinman RE, Greer FR, editors. Pediatric nutrition. 7th edition. Elk Grove Village (IL): American Academy of Pediatrics; 2014. p. 83–110.
2. Tsang R, editor. Nutrition of the preterm infant: scientific basis and practical guidelines. 2nd edition. Cincinnati (OH): Digital Educational Publishing; 2005.
3. Adamkin DH. Postdischarge nutritional therapy. J Perinatol 2006;26(Suppl 1): S27–30 [discussion: S31–3].
4. McLeod G, Sherriff J. Preventing postnatal growth failure–the significance of feeding when the preterm infant is clinically stable. Early Hum Dev 2007; 83(10):659–65.
5. Embleton NE, Pang N, Cooke RJ. Postnatal malnutrition and growth retardation: an inevitable consequence of current recommendations in preterm infants? Pediatrics 2001;107(2):270–3.
6. Lemons JA, Bauer CR, Oh W, et al. Very low birth weight outcomes of the National Institute of Child Health and Human Development Neonatal Research Network, January 1995 through December 1996. Pediatrics 2001;107(1):e1–8.
7. Dusick AM, Poindexter BB, Ehrenkranz RA, et al. Growth failure in the preterm infant: can we catch up? Semin Perinatol 2003;27(4):302–10.
8. Ehrenkranz RA, Dusick AM, Vohr BR, et al. Growth in the neonatal intensive care unit influences neurodevelopmental and growth outcomes of extremely low birth weight infants. Pediatrics 2006;117(4):1253–61.
9. Bhatia J. Post-discharge nutrition of preterm infants. J Perinatol 2005;25(Suppl 2): S15–6 [discussion: S17–8].
10. Steward DK. Growth outcomes of preterm infants in the neonatal intensive care unit: long-term considerations. Newborn Infant Nurs Rev 2012;12(4):214–20.
11. Ehrenkranz R, Younes N, Lemons JA, et al. Longitudinal growth of hospitalized very low birth weight infants. Pediatrics 1999;104(2):280–9.
12. Lucas A, Fewtrell MS, Morley R, et al. Randomized trial of nutrient-enriched formula versus standard formula for postdischarge preterm infants. Pediatrics 2001;108(3):703–11.
13. Cooke RJ. Catch-up growth: implications for the preterm and term infant. Eur J Clin Nutr 2010;64(Suppl 1):S8–10.
14. Ziegler ET, Carlson PJ, Carlson SJ. Aggressive nutrition of the very low birthweight infant. Clin Perinatol 2002;29:225–44.
15. Bhatia J, Griffin I, Anderson D, et al. Selected macro/micronutrient needs of the routine preterm infant. J Pediatr 2013;162(Suppl 3):S48–55.
16. Conrad A. Post-discharge nutrition for the preterm infant. J Neonatal Nurs 2013; 19(4):217–22.
17. Embleton ND. Optimal protein and energy intakes in preterm infants. Early Hum Dev 2007;83(12):831–7.
18. Tudehope D, Fewtrell M, Kashyap S, et al. Nutritional needs of the micropreterm infant. J Pediatr 2013;162(Suppl 3):S72–80.
19. American Academy of Pediatrics, Section on Breastfeeding. Breastfeeding and the use of human milk. Pediatrics 2012;129(3):e827–41.
20. Atkinson S. Human milk feeding of the Micropremie. Clin Perinatol 2000;27(1): 235–47.
21. Abrams SA. Committee on nutrition. Calcium and vitamin D requirements of enterally fed preterm infants. Pediatrics 2013;131(5):e1676–83.

22. Franz AR, Pohlandt F, Bode H, et al. Intrauterine, early neonatal, and postdischarge growth and neurodevelopmental outcome at 5.4 years in extremely preterm infants after intensive neonatal nutritional support. Pediatrics 2009;123(1): e101–9.

23. Shah MD, Shah SR. Nutrient deficiencies in the premature infant. Pediatr Clin North Am 2009;56(5):1069–83.

24. Lapillonne A, O'Connor DL, Wang D, et al. Nutritional recommendations for the late-preterm infant and the preterm infant after hospital discharge. J Pediatr 2013;162(Suppl 3):S90–100.

25. Poindexter BB, Schanler RJ. Enteral nutrition for the high-risk neonate. In: Gleason CA, Devaskar S, editors. Avery's Diseases of the Newborn. 9th edition. Philadelphia, PA: Elsevier Saunders; 2012. p. 952–62.

26. Cristofalo EA, Schanler RJ, Blanco CL, et al. Randomized trial of exclusive human milk versus preterm formula diets in extremely premature infants. J Pediatr 2013; 163(6):1592–5.e1.

27. Fewtrell M, Lucas A. Enteral feeding of the preterm infant. Curr Paediatr 2002; 12(2):98–103.

28. Schanler RJ. Outcomes of human milk-fed premature infants. Semin Perinatol 2011;35(1):29–33.

29. Greer FR. Post-discharge nutrition: what does the evidence support? Semin Perinatol 2007;31(2):89–95.

30. Bhatia J. Growth curves: how to best measure growth of the preterm infant. J Pediatr 2013;162(Suppl 3):S2–6.

31. Fenton TR, Kim JH. A systematic review and meta-analysis to revise the Fenton growth chart for preterm infants. BMC Pediatr 2013;13:59.

32. Olsen IE, Groveman SA, Lawson ML, et al. New intrauterine growth curves based on United States data. Pediatrics 2010;125(2):e214–24.

33. Hall RT. Nutritional follow-up of the breastfeeding premature infant after hospital discharge. Pediatr Clin North Am 2001;48(2):453–60.

34. Young L, Morgan J, McCormick FM, et al. Nutrient-enriched formula versus standard term formula for preterm infants following hospital discharge. Cochrane Database Syst Rev 2012;(3):CD004696.

35. Young L, Embleton ND, McCormick FM, et al. Multinutrient fortification of human breast milk for preterm infants following hospital discharge. Cochrane Database Syst Rev 2013;(2):CD004866.

36. O'Connor DL, Khan S, Weishuhn K, et al. Growth and nutrient intakes of human milk-fed preterm infants provided with extra energy and nutrients after hospital discharge. Pediatrics 2008;121(4):766–76.

37. O'Connor DL, Weishuhn K, Rovet J, et al. Visual development of human milk-fed preterm infants provided with extra energy and nutrients after hospital discharge. JPEN J Parenter Enteral Nutr 2012;36(3):349–53.

38. Leaf A, Subramanian S, Cherian S. Vitamins for preterm infants. Curr Paediatr 2004;14(4):298–305.

39. American Academy of Pediatrics Committee on Nutrition. Chapter 3: Breastfeeding. In: Kleinman RE, Greer F, editors. Pediatric nutrition. 7th edition. Elk Grove Village (IL): American Academy of Pediatrics; 2014. p. 42–3.

40. Rao R, Georgieff MK. Iron therapy for preterm infants. Clin Perinatol 2009;36(1): 27–42.

Index

Note: Page numbers of article titles are in **boldface** type.

Clin Perinatol 41 (2014) 475–485
http://dx.doi.org/10.1016/S0095-5108(14)00033-5   perinatology.theclinics.com
0095-5108/14/$ – see front matter © 2014 Elsevier Inc. All rights reserved.

Moving?

Make sure your subscription moves with you!

To notify us of your new address, find your **Clinics Account Number** (located on your mailing label above your name), and contact customer service at:

Email: journalscustomerservice-usa@elsevier.com

800-654-2452 (subscribers in the U.S. & Canada)
314-447-8871 (subscribers outside of the U.S. & Canada)

Fax number: 314-447-8029

Elsevier Health Sciences Division
Subscription Customer Service
3251 Riverport Lane
Maryland Heights, MO 63043

*To ensure uninterrupted delivery of your subscription, please notify us at least 4 weeks in advance of move.

ELSEVIER

SINGLETON HOSPITAL
STAFF LIBRARY